Medicine and Money

Physicians as Businessmen

Medicine and Money

Physicians as Businessmen

Joseph LaDou, M.D.
Woodside, California

James D. Likens, Ph.D.
Associate Professor of Economics
Pomona College
Claremont, California

Ballinger Publishing Company ● Cambridge, Massachusetts
A Subsidiary of J.B. Lippincott Company

R728
L28

Copyright © 1977 by Ballinger Publishing Company. All rights reserved. No part of this publication may be reproduced, stored in a retrieval system, or transmitted in any form or by any means, electronic, mechanical, photocopy, recording or otherwise, without the prior written consent of the publisher.

International Standard Book Number: 0-88410-145-2

Library of Congress Catalog Card Number: 77-2332

Printed in the United States of America

Library of Congress Cataloging in Publication Data

LaDou, Joseph.
   Medicine and Money.

   Includes bibliographical references.
   1. Medicine—Practice. 2. Medical economics—United States. 3. Physicians—United States. 4. Medical corporations—United States. I. Likens, James D., joint author. II. Title.
R728.L28   658.91′610973   77-2332
ISBN 0-88410-145-2

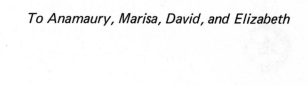

To Anamaury, Marisa, David, and Elizabeth

Contents

List of Figures

List of Tables

Acknowledgments

It is not possible to learn about the influence of physician behavior on the economics of health care delivery merely by studying published research findings. The virtual absence of a scholarly literature on some aspects of this topic led us to conduct extensive interviews with physicians, health administrators, accountants, and attorneys. This book would not have been possible without their help. In addition, many people with a wide diversity of professional backgrounds have given us their comments on various drafts of the book. The collective influence of these individuals on the final product is substantial indeed. We gratefully acknowledge the help and encouragement of all of these friends and associates, and especially the following: Milton Chatton, Roberta Clarke, Karlyn Cobb, Maxine Curtis, Jerry A. DiVecchio, Steven B. Epstein, Donald Heath, Michael E. Herbert, John C. Hershey, Frank M. Holden, David Jorgensen, Louise Moon, Ann A. Mothershead, George Pickett, Charles E. Phelps, Neill Piland, and Jack Rodgers. None of them, of course, should be blamed for the views we have expressed in this book or for any errors that may remain.

Rita Grigsby, Mary Lee Eubanks, Darlene Bolter, and Alice Jacobi provided much appreciated administrative and secretarial help to us.

Finally, we wish to acknowledge the invaluable editorial assistance of Mary I. Phares.

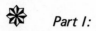 *Part I:*

Introduction

Introduction

Americans are engaged in a debate of great significance. At issue is the future role of the government in the delivery of health care. The debate is not a new one. For years, medical societies, health insurance companies, hospital associations, labor unions, consumer interest groups, government administrators, and politicians have argued about the form that the health care system should take. The intensity of the debate has increased in recent years, however, because fundamental decisions about health care are now being made at high political levels. The implications of these decisions for the future are enormous.

The most important product of this debate so far is likely to turn out to be a 1973 federal law to promote an alternative to the traditional fee-for-service medical system that currently dominates American medicine. This alternative is the Health Maintenance Organization (HMO). An HMO is comprised of a number of physicians from various medical specialties who provide for the total care of the patient. The most important innovation of HMOs is that, instead of paying for health services as they are provided, a family or individual pays the HMO for health care needs in advance with an annual premium, called a capitation fee. The HMOs are modeled on successful prepaid group practices such as the Kaiser Health Plan, which operates principally in the western United States. More than one hundred prepaid plans are now in operation, and the legislation will encourage their growth throughout the country in the hope that eventually almost every family in America will have access to the health care provided by such a plan.

Debate is also taking place about the role of government in financing health care. Numerous proposals for some form of national health insurance are currently before the Congress. Although they differ widely in scope and detail, all of these bills would provide new money for the purchase of medical services, and hence all of them could be expected to lead to an enlarged role for government in regulating the delivery of health care. Many observers have predicted that some form of national health insurance will soon be adopted. Indeed, such insurance might already be a reality if Congress had not been required to turn its attention away from health care legislation, first, by the Watergate scandals and, then, by the energy crisis and the accompanying inflation and recession. Whether these problems will create a long or only a short respite from dealing with the problems of health care, the political climate needed for serious congressional consideration of a national health insurance bill is bound to recur.

What forces have brought about this political debate to reform the present system of health care delivery? A partial list would include: (1) the difficulties created by advances in medical technology that not only add to the cost of medical care, but also force organizational change within medical institutions; (2) a belief by a large proportion of the population that quality health care should be the right of all citizens; (3) the enormous increase since World War II in the number of American families who pay for health care through private and public insurance; and (4) the widespread misconception that a shortage of physicians exists in the United States, which is reinforced by the existing geographical maldistribution of practitioners.

The combination of these forces has resulted in two serious criticisms of American health care. First, although American health care at its best is unsurpassed anywhere in the world, it is sometimes inadequate in terms of quantity and even in terms of quality. The American people spent $12 billion on health care in 1950, $26 billion in 1960, and $69 billion in 1970. By 1975, the amount spent had increased to more than $118 billion.[1] But, despite these large expenditures, many critics of American medicine claim that the country has not received its money's worth. To be sure, much of the money spent on health care was used to pay for the treatment of important acute and chronic medical problems, but a large part of it also went to pay for unnecessary medical care. Few dollars were used to promote preventive medicine or public health. And in spite of the existence of Medicare and Medicaid, many of the elderly and the poor receive inadequate medical attention, and health care in the inner cities and the rural areas is sometimes inadequate or non-existent.

Second, health care is expensive, and costs are spiralling every year. Per capita expenditures have increased from $78 in 1950 to $547 in 1975.[2] Although part of this increase has resulted from improvements in the quantity and quality of care being provided, a substantial share has gone to feed inflation in health care prices. Over the period 1950-1975, prices for all health care services increased by 225 percent and for hospitalization by more than 550 percent. The Consumer Price Index, by comparison, increased by 131 percent over this same period.[3] A sharp increase in health care prices occurred after 1966, when the Medicare and Medicaid programs infused new purchasing power into the health care system. In recent years, defensive medicine—medically unnecessary care provided by physicians to protect themselves in the event that they are accused in malpractice suits—has likely contributed substantially to the rise in medical prices. During the 1971-1974 price freeze, health care prices were contained somewhat; they increased by only 12.3 percent as compared with an 18.1 percent increase in the Consumer Price Index. With the removal of controls, however, they again climbed sharply: by 14 percent during the first year after controls were removed. Concurrently, the Consumer Price Index rose by much less—10 percent—even though the nation was involved in the "energy crisis." By the first quarter of 1976, the annual increase in the Consumer Price Index, less medical care, was slowed to 2.4 percent while overall health care prices were rising at an annual rate of 14.0 percent and hospital service charges were climbing at 20.1 percent per year.[4] Further increases in medical prices can be expected as the costs of large increases in malpractice insurance premiums are passed through the system to patients.

The authors of this book contend that the fundamental problems of health care delivery in the United States—high and rapidly rising costs and unnecessary care—stem mainly from three sources.

First, the typical physician is not trained to be a manager or a businessman. Yet, in his role as manager of an office-based practice—and most American physicians are office-based practitioners—the physician has a large and important managerial responsibility. He must plan for and organize a medical facility; hire, train, and supervise medical and support staff; purchase equipment; and establish procedures for managing a large volume of patients and paperwork. He must coordinate his practice with those of other physicians to obtain referrals, and he must interact with hospitals, laboratories, and private and public insurance companies. He is also asked to participate in the management of the hospital where he has staff privileges. The decisions he makes largely determine America's medical bill, because he is the center of the health care delivery system. But the typical physician is not inclined—either by disposition or by training—to be a manager. The consequence is a degree of inefficiency that costs the American people billions of dollars per year.

Second, the incentives in medical practice contribute to the social problems of unnecessary care and high and soaring health care costs. Even if physicians were effective business managers, the incentives that guide them would not encourage them to perform as society expects them to perform.

Third, the health care services field is not competitive. In a competitive business environment, if customers are not being served or served well, entrepreneurs in pursuit of profits will move in to offer a better product or superior service. If business firms are inefficient and their prices are too high, the pressures of competition will force them to become efficient and reduce their prices—or drive them out of the industry. But such is not the case in medicine. Physicians, since they are usually poor businessmen, seldom think in terms of cost effectiveness. Moreover, medical ethics, licensure laws, and regulations that prohibit advertising or the practice of medicine by business corporations discourage competition among physicians, reduce the effectiveness of the discipline of the marketplace, and make it difficult for competent nonphysician managers to rationalize health care organization. The result is a continuation of the nation's inefficient health care delivery system.

This book is about physicians as businessmen and the economic impact that they have on society. It begins with the physician, analyzing how society's expectations for its physicians, the methods used to recruit and train physicians, and the physician's personality combine to produce poor physician businessmen and an inefficient health care delivery system. Next, the economic incentives in health care delivery and the nature of competition in medicine are analyzed. The book ends with an examination of alternatives for reform. It concludes that attempts to reform health care delivery through nationalizaion, national health insurance, regulation, or HMOs—as these reforms are now conceived—will all fail because they do not effectively overcome the problems of poor management, perverse incentives, and inadequate competition. It also argues that increased participation by business corporations in health care delivery can strengthen management capability, modify incentives, and improve the social performance of the health care system.

Many books about physicians treat the physician either as a candidate for sainthood or as a selfish entrepreneur who is the easy target of the muckraker. Physicians in real life seldom fit either of these stereotypes. Consequently, this book is intended neither to honor nor condemn physicians. It is, rather, an attempt to observe the physician as he is and to examine his effect on the economics of health care.

❋   *Part II:*

The Economic Impact of the
Physician Businessman

Chapter Two

Physician Personality and Training

THE CASE OF "CHARLES DUDLEY WARNER, M.D."

Charles Dudley Warner, M.D.—45 years of age, board-certified specialist in internal medicine, past president of the local medical society—is at the peak of his medical career. *He is on the teaching staff of Community Hospital. His private practice is flourishing. His medical suite occupies a full floor in the city's newest office complex; the facility and equipment are the most advanced that technology can offer. Staffing this office are a registered nurse, a medical secretary, and a receptionist who doubles as a bookkeeper.*

Dr. Warner's personal life appears to be equally successful. He lives with his wife and three children in a $250,000 split-level brick house fronting on a river in a nearby "bedroom community." He owns three cars and a thirty-foot cabin cruiser and is a member of the golf and country club, an exclusive riding club, and the Symphony Association. Although he seldom has time to use the cabin cruiser, his two college-aged sons and seventeen-year-old daughter delight in cruising upriver with their friends. He also is rarely able to attend any of the functions of the social and cultural organizations to which he pays dues, but his wife frequently participates in their activities.

What spare time he has, Dr. Warner devotes to civic activities. He takes considerable pride in his community work, which has given him an identity in the community where he lives. His civic work, his medical background, and his affluent lifestyle have combined to give him an enviable position—admired by most and envied by many.

But, in fact, Dr. Warner has reached the lowest ebb in his life—financially, personally, and emotionally. In the past few months, he has even contemplated suicide.

At home, there are frequent arguments. His wife complains that he is never home, never takes her anywhere, and she must raise the children by herself. He complains that she spends too much on designer dresses, unnecessary folderol, and contributions to her favorite organizations. The arguments are never conclusive and usually end with their sleeping in separate rooms. Dr. Warner responds to these quarrels by throwing himself into his work, because he loves medicine and because his practice helps keep his mind off his problems.

His greatest concern is that he is deeply in debt. Only one of his cars (the five-year-old car that he drives to the office) is paid for. There is a very large mortgage on his home and payments to be made every month on the remaining cars and the cabin cruiser. He worries because he has not been able to save toward his retirement and is unable to take advantage of the tax-sheltering Keogh Plan because he does not have the funds to establish a retirement program for his three employees. He also worries about the $1,500-per-month rent on his medical suite, his high malpractice premiums, rising salaries for his staff, and loan payments on the furniture and equipment. His overhead is running close to 60 percent of his practice revenues and will probably rise to above 70 percent with the next increase in malpractice insurance premiums.

Two people have attempted to help Dr. Warner solve his financial problems. His accountant of many years, who knew more than anyone about the doctor's money problems, finally tried to counsel him about his business and personal finances. But the doctor viewed his accountant's suggestions as criticism and was stung by the implication that he was incapable of managing his own affairs. True, he often could not spend the proper time on his business and was forced to work on this aspect of his practice in the early hours of the morning. But then, that was the way a busy medical practice went. So he dismissed his accountant and found one who prepared financial statements and tax reports and offered no advice.

The attorney who had sent the Warners to a marriage counsellor a few years earlier also felt obligated to advise them financially. He recommended that they severely restrict their spending and seek the help of a top-flight financial counsellor. Dr. Warner received the advice without comment, but did not call on this particular attorney again.

Today, Dr. Warner is a middle-aged, debt-ridden, physically exhausted man who wonders what has happened to the bright promise he had expected when he graduated from medical school.

RECRUITING AND TRAINING OF PHYSICIANS

The financial and business problems that "Dr. Warner" and many other physicians face are rooted far back in their medical careers. Many of their problems begin during the premedical period and in medical school. Some are of even longer standing and derive from the attitudes of society toward its physicians, attitudes acquired as much from television stereotypes and fantasy as from real life.

In industrialized countries, the young men and women who enter medicine are carefully selected from among the highest academic achievers and the strongest physical specimens. Society impresses on them that medicine is an exalted profession and that those who enter it should be both gifted and dedicated. Thus, they enter medical school recognized as achievers and secure in the belief that they are a special breed. By the time they graduate, they are convinced that they are on the brink of an outstanding and fulfilling life.

The American Medical Association, in its handbook entitled *Horizons Unlimited,* counsels these young men and women that "the student who really wants to enter medicine and goes on to earn his M.D. degree will forever be compensated for any sacrifices he has made and any hardships he has endured by the immense self-satisfaction which comes from saving the lives and alleviating the pain and suffering of his patients." After a discussion of the respect that physicians merit and their earnings potential, it cautions that "the student who selects medicine as his career choice should not, however, be swayed by a mere desire to enjoy its potential, superficial merits—prestige, glamor, or financial rewards. He should be motivated primarily by a desire to help his fellow man and contribute to the increasing progress of medicine."[1]

The Premedical Influence
Acceptance into medical school is greeted by the premedical student, his family, and his peers with as much pride and satisfaction as is shown for any other accomplishments in our educational system. But this success is achieved only after completing a highly intensive and competitive course of study at the undergraduate level. In this environment, the premedical student must become achievement oriented—that is to say, grades oriented. As shown by Table 2-1, he or she will devote the major portion of study time to the

Table 2-1. Summary of Required Premedical Subjects

Required Courses	Percentage of Courses Required by Medical Schools
Biology (comparative anatomy, embryology, zoology, genetics)	20%
Chemistry (inorganic, organic, physical chemistry, quantitative analysis, qualitative analysis)	36%
Physics	15%
Mathematics (analytical geometry, calculus, trigonometry)	11%
Humanities (English, language, literature)	16%
Social and behavioral sciences	2%
	100%

Source: Calculated from V. L. Wilson, ed., *Medical School Admission Requirements, 1975-76, U.S.A. and Canada* (Washington, D.C.: Association of American Medical Colleges, 1974), p. 3.

sciences, and at the same time, must meet only a minimal requirement for liberal arts studies.

The Association of American Medical Colleges, in its *Directory of Medical School Admission Requirements*, states that:

> A major function of the liberal arts college is to aid in the development of perceptive, knowledgeable citizens. The total experience provided by the college should facilitate understanding and the acquisition of intellectual patterns that could be employed in a variety of fields including medicine. Medicine needs individuals with a diversity of educational backgrounds and a wide variety of talents and interests. The philosophies of education, specific premedical course requirements, other qualifications for enrollment, and systems of training vary among the medical schools, but all recognize the desirability of a broad education—a good foundation in the natural sciences (mathematics, chemistry, biology, and physics), highly developed communication skills, and a solid background in the social sciences and humanities.[2]

A "broad education" for premedical students would include not only science courses, but also humanities, social sciences, economics, and perhaps business administration. Despite the rhetoric recommending a "broad education," medical school admissions committees appear to attach little importance to the liberal arts. The result is that courses in the basic sciences monopolize the time and commitment of the premedical student. Because of the emphasis on science courses and the great amount of time that these courses consume, students commonly meet their liberal arts requirements with courses that will yield the highest grades for the least effort. Consequently, the matriculating student may be academically acceptable to a medical school but otherwise intellectually underdeveloped.

Table 2-2.   Medical School Application Activity

First-Year Class	Number of Applicants	No. of Accepted Applicants	Percentage Accepted Applicants
1970-71	24,987	11,500	46.0
1971-72	29,172	12,335	42.3
1972-73	36,135	13,757	38.1
1973-74	40,506	14,335	35.4
1974-75	42,624	15,066	35.3
1975-76	42,303	15,365	36.3

Source: Statistics for 1970-1971 through 1974-75 are from A. E. Crowley, ed., "Medical Education in the United States 1974-75," *Journal of the American Medical Association,* vol. 234, no. 13 (December 1975), p. 1337. Data for 1975-76 are preliminary estimates of the Association of American Medical Colleges.

The competition for medical school admission is intense. Although medical schools are increasing in number and size, Table 2-2 shows that many more students are applying than can be accepted. Many educators familiar with medical school admissions say that, of all students applying to medical school, probably two-thirds are qualified to become good physicians. Yet only slightly more than one-third are now being accepted.

A number of medical educators have expressed alarm over the emergence of large numbers of students who are so achievement-oriented that their only goal at the undergraduate level is to be accepted into medical school.[3] Psychiatrists have noted that the system selects those students for medical school who do best in their examinations, who are interested in the physical sciences, and inadvertently, who are generally conventional and prone to emotional inhibition, rather than the unconventional who are more likely to have an interest in people and to be uninhibited emotionally.[4]

The Impact of Medical School

Two types of physicians teach medicine: academicians and practicing physicians. The full-time academicians devote their efforts to
research as well as teaching. They typically lack private practice
experience and probably would not consider medical office management a topic worthy of study or discussion. The private practitioners,
who teach on a part-time basis, are unstinting in sharing their clinical
knowledge and experience, but they rarely mention their experience
in office management or discuss the business aspects of medical
practice. The private practitioner obviously employs a staff, bills his
patients for services rendered, and derives an income sufficient to
support his family and himself, but the student is not given the
vaguest understanding of how a medical business is managed. Unfortunately, even if they were so inclined, most private practitioners
would be unable to tell the student how to operate effectively the
business of a medical practice.

For the vast majority of medical students, these business considerations are of only minor importance. They still face a year of intern-
ship prior to full medical licensure. Furthermore, there is a choice
to be made between general practice, family practice (which requires
further clinical training), or a residency program to become a specialist in one of medicine's many fields of special endeavor, such as
internal medicine or pediatrics (typically two or three years of
further training), or general surgery and other surgical areas (usually
four to six years of further training). Again, during these long periods
of training, little or no mention is made of medical business management.

Taking a cue from his teachers, the young trainee devotes his
entire attention to patient care to the exclusion of any interest in
practice management. This pattern will most likely continue throughout his professional career.

A PROFILE OF THE PHYSICIAN

Students who enter the medical profession tend to be the eldest or
only child in a family. Thus, they tend to fit the known profile of
first and only children—that is, they are serious, responsible, con-
forming, compulsive, authoritarian, and successful, but not necessarily satisfied with themselves or happier than their peers.[5] The
preponderance also tend to have a compulsive drive to be accepted
into the medical profession.

Psychiatric studies of medical students characterized as "normal"
or "successful" have been summarized as follows:

These students are usually obsessive, compulsive, orderly, highly organized, responding to the dictates of their own conscience. Their modes of functioning are rather basic attributes of what are called a "healthy" obsessive compulsive character. That is, productivity, achievement, isolation, denial, and repression serve to protect the student from disturbing intrapsychic and interpersonal conflicts. They tend to strive for mastery, control, and thoroughness along with safety and self-restraint. They put intellectual matters above emotions, security above pleasure, service to others above self-service, exactitude above fantasy. They work harder than most for good grades in subjects they care little about. Faculty members describe the typical medical student as a hard worker, extremely conscientious, a little shy and retiring, who doesn't let go of his feelings, and is somewhat hard to draw out. They have a balance between active and passive characteristics, indicating that there is an ability to shift defenses as the occasion arises. They suppress their aggressive and sexual impulses in the interest of satisfying conscience and need for security. Admission committees tend to select this type either because of a preference for this character or because of a preponderance of these students among the applicants. At any rate it is the self-disciplined and conscientious student who finds the going easier and who seems to adjust better to the stringent demands of the medical curriculum.[6]

Historically, the typical applicant accepted into medical school has been a male with an outstanding academic record and good health. Few women were accepted in the past regardless of their academic achievements or state of health. This pattern, however, has been changing steadily over the past several years. In 1939, 5.0 percent of the students entering medical schools were women, as compared with 11.1 in 1970 and 22.3 percent in 1974. Today, most medical schools are eager to enroll qualified young women. Of the 1975 medical school graduates, 13.4 percent were women, which represents the highest number and the highest proportion in history.[7]

The 1960s and 1970s have also seen a rise in the number of students of ethnic minorities who are accepted into medical schools. (Minority enrollment statistics were instituted in 1960.) The minority group students doubled in numbers between school year 1969-70 and 1974-75 from 4.2 to 8.8 percent.[8]

In recent years, foreign medical graduates have become a substantial fraction of the nation's physicians. About one-fifth of all practicing physicians and nearly one-third of those in internships and residencies in the United States are foreign medical graduates.[9] These physicians tend to be hospital-based rather than office-based, patient care physicians: In 1974 foreign medical graduates constituted 32.0 percent of the former category and 13.5 percent of the latter.[10] To date they are concentrated in a few states, with one-fourth being located in New York, and one-half being situated in that state plus Illinois, Ohio, New Jersey, and California.[11] Foreign medical graduates constitute one-third or more of the physician populations of Delaware, Illinois, New Jersey, New York, and Rhode Island.[12]

In the 1967–68 school year, 20 percent of U.S. medical students came from families with incomes of $25,000 or more per year; the median was $13,010 compared with $7,973 for the population as a whole. However, 25 percent came from families having annual incomes of less than $5,000, 20 percent from families where the father held a blue-collar job, and 33 percent from families in which the head of the household had not graduated from high school.[13] Students from low- and middle-income families are able to attend medical school because of the availability of loan funds from many sources, including medical schools, the federally sponsored Health Professions Scholarship Program, and various grants-in-aid and tuition-remission grants.

As a result of the high cost of medical school and the ready availability of loan funds, the average medical student is in debt long before he or she graduates. In 1966, 54.3 percent of the students in 94 medical schools borrowed approximately $20 million in long-term, low-interest loans through their medical schools. In 1975, a similar percentage of students borrowed or received aid in excess of $50 million.[14] Some evidence indicates that the actual proportion of students who go into debt is much greater than indicated by these figures derived from questionnaire surveys.

During the entire course of study that produces a physician, the married medical trainee has little time to develop a wholesome family life. Many medical families soon establish a pattern of limited personal interaction between the physician and other family members. Unfortunately, this situation seldom improves over time.

Many young women see that physicians' families live in expensive houses, drive good cars, and offer their children many of the advantages associated with high-income brackets. The idea of marrying a medical student or young physician and helping him in his important mission is also appealing to a young woman. The young medical wife often makes the same basic assumption about her husband's earning potential as he does—that is, there may be some sacrifices, but there will always be financial security. She is as naive as he about the ultimate price to be paid for financial success. The "jealous mistress" of medicine will consume much of her husband's thoughts and energies all of his working life. The high income they anticipated will come only from working very long hours. Little opportunity will be left to enjoy life or to ease his frenzied pace.

James L. Evans, a psychiatrist, has examined the personalities and symptoms of doctors' wives who were hospitalized for psychiatric illness. Depression was their common complaint. He suggests that a number of these women married doctors because they wanted husbands who would provide an unusual degree of understanding and protection within the marital relationship. When their idealized father/doctor image collapses because the doctor has become increasingly involved in the demands generated by his work and his patients, they become emotionally ill. Evans emphasizes one problem that is the subject of frequent jokes at medical cocktail parties; so frequent, in fact, that we can be fairly certain that it is a real and serious issue in medical marriages. Evans puts it thus:

> The physician, secure in his omnipotent role with patients who are frankly dependent upon his professional capabilities, rejected his wife's dependency strivings except when they were expressed as demands for "medical" attention. He then, without apparent cognizance of their emotional basis, gratified these needs by resorting to his professional role. How often do we hear the pretty wife's complaint "Of course, to get any real time or attention from my husband I need to book an appointment through his secretary."[15]

Although the high rate of divorce among physicians is not alarming by today's standards, the incidence of informal and legal separation is. The practice of medicine offers a ready-made excuse to retreat from the difficulties of marriage. Who can criticize the physician for working so hard at his practice? Who can fault his wife for wanting her husband not to drive himself so hard? Ultimately, many medical wives decide that they can enjoy their husband's earnings just as well with a separation or divorce as they can with his occasionally dropping by the house in a state of fatigue, bringing with him concerns about his patients and his office.

Few courts direct the physician's wife to support herself after dissolution of a marriage. The judge is likely to make the same basic assumption about physicians' earning power as do most lay people. He is also likely to realize that the sense of responsibility inherent in the physician personality will cause him to accept without complaint long periods of alimony payment and generous child support, even if not stipulated by court decree.

The operation and management of a medical practice can take a tremendous toll—both physically and emotionally—on the physician. The effects are usually not evident until after age forty-five. Up to that time, physicians have a lower death rate than other people, although their longevity is almost identical with that of the population as a whole. The stronger performance of physicians in their earlier years very likely reflects the superior physical condition required of medical school applicants. After age forty-five, however, physicians have a higher death rate than the general population, with the primary cause of death being cardiovascular disease.[16] Thus, many of them, like "Dr. Warner," reach their lowest point—physically, emotionally, and financially—at an age when men in other fields of endeavor are at the peak of their capabilities.

Because of their proclivity, as a group, for cardiovascular diseases, physicians have been studied with regard to their personality types. This typing of physician personality is the result of recent interest in Type A and Type B personalities as they relate to heart disease. The Type A person has been determined to be a successful, hyperconscientious, ambitious, hard-driving, time-oriented individual. The Type B personality, on the other hand, is antithetical; he may be equally successful, but he approaches life in a more easy-going, less stressful manner. Type As have been reported to have a higher prevalence of coronary disease than Type Bs. An "average" man is scored 0 in all of these attributes, persons tending toward Type A are given positive values, and those in Type B score negative values. Physicians were conclusively "Super As" (mean score, +5.5; highest means score previously recorded for a group of professional men, +5.3). Physicians ranked among the most impatient of people (mean score, +4.4; the highest mean impatience score previously recorded, +4.6).[17]

The average work week of many physicians is more than fifty hours.[18] Add to that, the hours spent tied to the telephone, while on call, as well as the ringing telephone during the night that interrupts sleep and contributes to the fatigue of the next long day. The "responsible" trait of physicians precludes complaining. Indeed, most physicians take pride in their intense devotion to their practices. Rising before the family awakens to make hospital rounds, snacking between patient visits rather than relaxing with a meal, and working into the night are the rule, not the exception, for most medical practitioners. Because the physician is convinced that this approach is best for his patients, he does not question the long hours of work. Little time is left for exercise, leisure, and the enjoyment of his family. As likely as not, when he recommends preventive medicine by discussing exercise, weight control, and leisure-time activities with his patients, he is less than a model to them.

The stress of medical practice has been presumed to explain the alarming rate of suicide, drug and alcohol addiction, and failure in marriage among physicians. The doctor's compulsive personality might also explain the frustration and depression that precede suicide. For the general population, the suicide rate is 10.5/100,000. The rate reported for physicians is at least 33/100,000 ranging between 12/100,000 for radiologists and 70/100,000 for psychiatrists.[19] Approximately one hundred physicians are reported to commit suicide each year in the United States, and the actual number is undoubtedly higher. One hundred physician suicides is equivalent to an entire graduating class of the average medical school. And most are under age fifty—in the middle of their most productive years.[20]

The rate of alcoholism and drug addiction is also high among physicians. With regard to narcotics, physicians as a group have an alarming incidence of addiction, ranging from 1/100 to 1/400. Thirty to one hundred times as many physicians suffer from drug dependency as does the general population, with Demerol being the narcotic most frequently abused. Drug addiction is an occupational hazard because of the physician's ready access to drugs. The incidence of alcoholism is not accurately known, but all indications are that it far surpasses the rate of the general population.[21] There is an old bit of humor that says "The physician's diagnosis of an alcoholic is the person who drinks more than he does." Clearly, the incidence of broken marriages, suicide, and drug and alcohol misuse are only symptoms of many physicians' inability to cope with the unrelenting stresses of medical practice.

Studies have shown that doctors demonstrate a higher level of anxiety than persons in other fields and that practicing physicians exhibit higher anxiety levels than physicians engaged in research and administration.[22] They are especially troubled by the management of chronic, frustrating cases and the death of patients, particularly children and adolescents.

Overwork can be interpreted as a mechanism of retreat from overwhelming personal conflict. Often when good sense and sound personal hygiene clearly indicate the need for a doctor to slow down, he will enter into a form of maladaptive behavior. By working irregular hours, working inefficiently, sleeping and eating only sporadically, he will tend to withdraw from family responsibilities and begin to experience unaccustomed difficulties in the management of his patients and to show a reluctance to refer those patients elsewhere for fear of loss of face.

In view of the serious effects of stress on physicians, surprisingly few studies have been conducted about this problem. Some few studies have looked in depth at those physicians who have encountered personal or professional problems that have required clinical intervention. In these extreme cases, basic insecurity and vulnerability is clearly identified and is often accompanied by a highly ambivalent attitude toward medicine—loving it, yet resenting its continuing demands—because it fails to meet personal needs.[23] But little research has investigated the effect of stress on physicians in general.

Physician personalities, however, have been carefully analyzed. George E. Vaillant and his associates studied a group of people who were initially selected during their college years. The group included forty-five students who eventually became doctors. The study findings revealed that these physicians were statistically more likely than people who chose other occupations to show traits of dependency, pessimism, passivity, and self-doubt. They were also found to be more inclined to exhibit feelings of anger against themselves rather than to act it out.[24] Another study of eight hundred gifted men confirmed that feelings of inferiority are more common among physicians than among the general population.[25] From these studies, some researchers have concluded that the physician personality is as important as stress in explaining why physicians are more likely than other people to have unsuccessful marriages, to use alcohol and drugs heavily, and to require psychotherapy.

MOTIVATIONS FOR BECOMING A PHYSICIAN

Studies of the occupational choice of college students show that premedical students have a high regard for the "opportunity to be helpful to others." However, they also want to earn a great deal of money and to obtain social status and prestige.[26] This diverse combination of goals caused the author of one study to conclude that prospective physicians demonstrate a "curious ideological ambivalence, composed in part of an inclination to assume a service orientation in the form of wishing to help people, but countered by an inclination to desire prestige and money as well."[27] The author notes that the desire to help people is supposed to be characteristic of the physician, while the desire to earn profits is more characteristic of the businessman. This expectation may be a reflection of the public's wish that physicians be selfless servants of society. If so, the expectation is misplaced. Both business students and premedical students are motivated to earn money.

In a nationwide personal interview survey undertaken in 1956, the year "Dr. Warner" graduated from medical school, 1,086 male medical students ranked "the opportunity to work with people" as the most important goal of their future careers in medicine.[28]

Financial gain, social position, and opportunity to conduct scientific research were considered secondary objectives, although income was rated relatively high as a goal.

Despite these findings, there are important differences between traditional businessmen and physicians. Although both seek success and recognition, they define their goals differently. The business-man's concept of success emphasizes high income and social prestige in the community. The physician's concept of success includes these values, but also stresses professional aspirations—achieving a high degree of technical competence, adhering to the norms of service and autonomy, and earning the respect of patients and colleagues.

The goals of the physician have been identified by John Colombotos of Columbia University. In interviews with 1,142 male private practitioners in New York State Colombotos asked the following questions:[29]

Which of the following things was the most important to you in your decision to go into medicine—was it the social prestige of a medi-cal career, the chance to help people, the chance to do work of special interest to you, or the economic opportunity?

Which of these things was second most important to you in your decision to go into medicine?

What about the present—which of these things is most important to you now—is it the social prestige of a medical career . . .?

Which of these things is second most important to you now?

Results of the survey indicate that physicians from lower-income backgrounds were much more likely than those from upper-income backgrounds to stress success values (i.e., either economic oppor-tunity or social prestige or both) as reasons for going into medicine. More than half of the respondents (55 percent) in the lowest socio-economic category were success oriented, compared with 22 percent in this group whose fathers were physicians. When asked about their present concern with economic success and social prestige, however, all groups reported that these factors are no longer as important. Colombotos interpreted this reported reduction in emphasis on money and prestige as stemming from two causes.

First, although money and prestige are "important" to many people in selecting a career in medicine—particularly to persons from lower-income backgrounds—these goals become less "important" once they are achieved. Second, socialization brought about by con-tact with professional colleagues may contribute to the change. Although socioeconomic background has a strong influence on a person's reasons for entering medicine, teachers and colleagues eventually modify the effects of earlier influences. The more success-oriented become less so, and the less success-oriented become more so.

EARLY BUSINESS DECISIONS

Attention has thus far been focused on factors that contribute to the poor performance of physicians in their role as business managers— that is, educational background and psychological makeup. Among the consequences of these factors—the stringent emphasis of the medical schools on the healing arts, the lack of training in business decision making, and restrictive personality traits that are fairly com-mon among those entering the medical profession—is that frequently the beginning physician acts unwisely when choosing his area of specialization, location of practice, and type of practice mode.

Specialization

A longitudinal study sponsored by the National Institutes of Health indicates that the choice of specialty training made by most medical school graduates is largely predictable on the basis of per-sonality characteristics.[30] Pragmatic considerations, such as the consumer demand in various communities for certain types of medical specialists, appear to play only a minor role in the selection of a medical specialty.

There are no agencies or counselling services that direct young physicians into specialty training based on the requirements of the population in any given area. Nor does the fact that such help is needed appear to occur to these entering doctors. Most of them assume that all areas of medicine are both lucrative and needed by society. But this assumption is not supported by fact.

For instance, there is an abundance of general surgeons in the United States, and various surgical subspecialties are in more than adequate supply as well. In some areas, pediatricians and obstetri-cians have been hard hit by the decline in the birth rate. Psychia-trists are being displaced by psychologists and therapists who are without medical background, but who are fully competent to handle problems not requiring drug treatment. At the same time, the country is faced with a decline in the number of general practitioners. During the period between 1963 and 1973, the number of specialists increased by 43.7 percent while the number of general practitioners declined by 26.6 percent.[31]

Thus, as is typical of many physician decisions, the choice of a specialty is often made with very little thought given to the business implications of that choice.

Location of the Practice

Most U.S. physicians are urban-reared and trained, and consequently choose to locate their practices in urban areas. In deciding where to locate, most doctors are also influenced strongly by climatic and geographic features and by the opportunity for contact with other physicians, as well as by the availability of clinical support facilities, medical schools and medical centers, and recreational and sports facilities.[32] The income status of physicians in the chosen area apparently is less important than the foregoing considerations. The physician's first business decision—where to locate his practice—is typically based not on economic realities but on his belief that his practice will succeed wherever he decides to establish it. Just as the pediatric or obstetric resident may fail to consider that improved birth control methods and a heightened social interest in population control will diminish the demand for his service, so the physician, regardless of specialty, tends to locate his practice with little concern for the economic factors that could dominate his entire professional life.

Physicians are inclined not only to locate in urban areas, but also to prefer certain states—particularly California and Florida. California retains 76.3 percent of the graduates of its medical schools and Florida, 53.1 percent. These states also attract large numbers of medical school graduates from other states. Migrating graduates constitute 72.3 percent of the physician population in California and 93 percent in Florida. At the same time, states such as Louisiana, Tennessee, Nebraska, and Vermont are faced with a shortage of physicians despite their steadily increasing numbers of medical school graduates.[33]

The decisions of the majority of physicians to establish their practices in the highly competitive urban areas of states that offer attractive living conditions show little concern for the needs of the population. Moreover, often the physician is not aware that physician incomes are frequently lower in the most attractive urban locales.

The Dream and the Reality

All too frequently, the dreams of the medical student of enjoying a rewarding, productive, and lucrative career are shattered by his practice experience. Often he finds in middle age that his rewards are overwork, fatigue, and impaired health, and in many cases, failure in marriage, and, sometimes, even drug and alcohol dependence, and suicide. Like Dr. Warner, many physicians in their middle years may ask—has it been worth it? Certainly, helping the ill and injured is a source of great satisfaction. But how many physicians grow weary of the sheer patient volume required to support the high overhead of a practice? How many, in the face of broken marriages and financial problems, begin to resent the demands of their profession? All too often the disappointment comes because the reality of medical practice differs so radically from the young doctor's dream.

Chapter Three

The Physician Businessman

STARTING THE MEDICAL PRACTICE

The physician normally trains in a large hospital. The hospital becomes his home while he is in training. It provides meals, laundry service, on-duty sleeping quarters, and often, total living accommodations. The fact that so many of the needs of the student, intern, or resident are taken care of by others in this environment suggests one reason that he is so unprepared for what lies ahead. Moreover, physician instructors and faculty seldom discuss—and are almost never asked to describe—the realities of medical practice. Thus, the physician going into private practice is unprepared for the real world of traditional business values and practices that he must enter. Most physicians recall this transition as the most trying experience in their professional lives.

Operating a practice effectively will require a business sense the physician most likely does not possess. He does not know how to plan and organize an effective office system or how to hire and supervise people. He probably cannot interpret a financial statement, let alone provide good financial management for his practice.

Although he is the product of the best medical education in the world, the beginning physician is virtually ignorant of the business reality that lies ahead. As he is unprepared for establishing and managing a medical practice, so is he unaware of the other problems that will beset him: the struggle for patients, the constraints that medicine will place on his family life, and the physical and emotional demands that medicine will make of him.

27

Just as the physician has given little thought to running a business, he has probably never pictured himself marketing his services. In fact, his actively seeking patients is "unethical," and the medical profession is proud of its record in maintaining the ethic of non-solicitation among physicians.

But to establish a practice, the physician must generate a flow of patients. Toward this end, his wife and her social contacts can serve in an important public relations function. Members of her clubs and other social acquaintances are of inestimable value in introducing new patients to the husband's practice. In his initial efforts to become known in the community, the physician may also participate in service clubs and scouting groups—probably for the only time in his working life. Most important, his contact with other physicians at the hospital and during hospital staff meetings are crucial if the young specialist is to receive patients on referral from other doctors. At such meetings, as well as in social encounters, he must bring referring physicians up to date on his care of their patients. In addition to demonstrating medical competence, he must express appreciation for all referrals. Country clubs, which provide a good atmosphere for interchange with other doctors, thrive on physician family memberships.

CLERICAL CHAOS IN THE MEDICAL OFFICE

With the flow of patients come the problems of office management: cash flow, billing and accounting, maintaining of accurate medical records, and dozens of other considerations. Only now does the physician begin to realize his lack of preparation for operating an efficient medical office. Because of his training and personality, he wishes to be in total control of his practice. However, the most common complaint among medical office personnel is that the doctor will not provide the guidance they need to solve their office problems. Often he does not understand much of what goes on in his business office and could not possibly learn in the time available between patient visits. But he does not want to appear ignorant of how to solve the problems of managing a business, and he does not want to appear overly interested in money. He may conclude, therefore, that greater cash volume will yield an income large enough to offset the lack of office efficiency. So he concentrates on seeing more patients rather than on improving office procedures. Unfortunately, more patients only add to office inefficiency.

As in any business, a well-managed medical office requires systemization of patient care and paperwork. Establishing a routine is not easy in medical practice. The physician's system of patient care is often unavoidably disrupted, usually by a medical emergency, and too often he carries this crisis approach into the clerical side of his practice as well. With little regard for the importance of the systemization of paperwork and with no clear understanding of the time required to accomplish various activities, he often decides what must be done according to the pressures of the moment, rather than by following well-established procedures.

Another common management failing is a tendency for the physician to pay premium salaries to his medical personnel while at the same time failing to acquire qualified clerical help. Having made this mistake, he compounds the problem by not using the talents in his office staff appropriately. For example, he may ask a highly paid nurse to run an errand, while relying on a lower paid secretary to establish a billing system whose inefficiency will cost his office large sums of money in the ensuing years.

Wages and salaries far outweigh the costs of capital equipment and office space in the daily operation of the medical office.[1] To minimize labor-related costs, the physician characteristically hires low-salaried clerical workers who must be trained on the job. But he seldom knows how to train them. If he pirates away experienced personnel from another physician, they will bring with them all the inefficiencies of their former employer's office. Unfortunately, few programs exist in the United States for training clerical personnel to support a medical practice.

Furthermore, the complexities of billing and accounting--numerous insurance company forms, government program forms, and required reports—have made using nurses or nursing assistants to double as clerical help all but impossible. Trained clerical personnel are vital to the physician, but typically he does not know how to select them and cannot adequately evaluate their work once they are employed. However, although medical personnel can seldom do clerical work, utilization of clerical staff to do medical work can be a cost-effective way to handle busy periods in the office. But seldom does the physician follow this course.

The physician is unusual who is willing to pay wages high enough to attract and keep competent clerical workers. Consequently, inefficiency is rampant in the medical office. The physician, although he is a master of detail, seldom understands or monitors all the business activities of his practice. But he desires the security of an orderly office where he believes himself to be in charge and where the needs of his patients are given foremost priority. Consequently, he must rely on an office staff that soon learns that the best way to keep him happy is to have all things appear to be in order. The underlying chaos is not apparent to the doctor; it would be apparent only to an accountant.

Office chaos often leads to intervention by the helpful wife. Although nothing lowers office morale and spurs employee turnover like the medical wife in the business office, wives are answering the phones and balancing the books of thousands of medical practices across the country. Physicians and their wives sitting down at the end of a busy day to type the numerous payment claims forms and medical dictation that have accumulated is not unusual. Doctors offer a number of explanations for this poor utilization of their scarce time. The most common justification is that they "seem to feel better knowing that everything is done correctly."

The physician's sensitivity to the feelings of others may lead his staff to abuse office privileges. In many instances he is so sensitive to his employees' personal problems that he gives them more time away from his office for illness and emergencies than is justifiable. Employee absences are a common problem in medical offices, and such absences can be counted in inefficiency and added costs.

A problem that sometime contributes to inefficiency in the group practice office is the individual physician's demand that systems be developed to meet his individual needs. A typical example occurs when a new partner is added to a small association or group medical practice. His concern for his patients causes him to demand immediate availability of patient records, x-ray reports, and other clerical information for each of his cases. To satisfy his demands, the office may duplicate personnel and equipment rather than insist that the new physician utilize the office system already in operation. As a result, the group can easily become a pyramid of solo practices and miss the efficiencies possible in a group practice with a centralized business office. The solution to this problem is to employ an office manager who will stand up to the physician whose demands are, of course, "always in the patient's best interest."

Finally, the inefficient billing of patients creates more chaos. Virtually all physicians dislike the fee aspects of treating patients and feel that money detracts from their relationship with their patients. Physicians often do not charge for fully delivered services or supplies because they fail to note them properly on a billing slip. Various medical billing services estimate that this inadvertent, but consistent, error results in a 10–20 percent loss in medical revenues.

Charges for services also can result in feelings of resentment on both sides and occasional bursts of anger on the part of the patient.

Doctors are wounded by angry letters and phone calls from patients complaining about charges. Consequently, physicians are slow to demand payment. Using a collection agency embarrasses them, and many county medical societies still consider such demands unethical. The fact that acceptance of charge cards is widely debated in medical circles further demonstrates the embarrassment doctors experience in trading their services for money. When no longer required to bill patients, as occurs when physicians begin to work in contractual medical practices, military, or company employment, many doctors express great relief.

When asked about the efficiency of physician offices, one accountant who specializes in physician practices replied, "I would say that only 25 percent of medical offices are well run. Another 25 percent are operating satisfactorily, but need improvement. Still another 25 percent need a great deal of improvement before they will be well-run. The remaining 25 percent are in a complete state of chaos. The inefficiencies of medical offices and the financial loss to the physician and his patients are simply unbelievable." This is a typical finding of accountants who specialize in medical practice accounting.

THE PHYSICIAN AS A MONEY MANAGER

Although only meager data are available concerning the money management habits of physicians, the authors' numerous interviews with knowledgeable financial managers indicate a single conclusion. Most physicians are poor money managers. They enter practice educationally unprepared to handle their financial futures.

Personal Finance

Doctors typically begin earning a living later than do businessmen and other professionals. Because of the high cost of medical education, most young physicians enter medicine with a diploma and some degree of indebtedness. Many enter the profession with an indebtedness as high as $30,000. Furthermore, during their educational period, they—and their families if they were married—were on very restricted incomes and lived "like students." Consequently, they eagerly anticipate the full life that they have been led to expect will come with medical practice.

Their wives and children may also be expected to have financial aspirations. Private schools, expensive cars, homes in affluent neighborhoods, and memberships in country clubs are the cultural goals of many physicians' families. A home in a middle-income neighborhood is often considered to be only temporary, because the doctor's family believes that, ultimately, the success of his medical practice will take them to affluent surroundings Even his patients may expect the doctor to achieve these goals to demonstrate his success and competence in medical practice. Often in their eagerness to begin the good life, the physician and his family become the victims of financial overcommitment.

Consider the financial experience of one young physcian entering practice in an urban area of Colorado. This young man came out of medical school and residency training owing $25,000 borrowed to finance his education. His accountant tells the story: "The man across the desk from me was a superbly trained medical man. Four years of college, then four years of medical school, one of internship, and three in residency had made him a master of his profession —and as helpless as a newborn babe when it came to business. Twelve years of study and training had produced a specialist in medicine. Those twelve years saw him lead an isolated, concentrated existence that scarcely allowed time for a minimal personal life, to say nothing of practical, everyday business affairs. The irony is that these remarkable specialists make, generally speaking, enormous incomes. And yet, nothing in their training prepares them for the management of those great sums of money."

An insurance agent convinced the young doctor and his wife to purchase a $400,000 insurance policy when $100,000 would probably have provided adequate coverage. To pay for the policy, the agent also arranged a $10,000 bank loan for him that made it unnecessary to pay premiums for the first four years. The physician signed a four-year, 6¾ percent note, allowing the bank to hold the policy as security.

The young physician then took out a loan of $30,000 to establish his practice. Of this sum, $20,000 was earmarked for office expenses and the remaining $10,000 for living expenses. The bank was helpful and allowed him to sign a seven-year note at 7 percent interest. During those seven years, all he had to pay was the interest, which amounted to a mere $210 a year. At the end of the seven years, as was explained to him, he could pay back the entire loan from the income he would accumulate from his practice. Another bank financed the purchase of a car with a small loan of $4,000 at 7¼ percent interest and easy monthly payments. A fourth bank advanced $50,000 at 7¾ percent for the purchase of a modest house in the vicinity of his practice.

Because the young doctor was an excellent physician, he began to generate $3,000 in monthly net revenue almost from the beginning. An anticipated $36,000 pretax income was heady success for two young people who had lived without much money most of their lives.

Among their assets, aside from the practice, were their home ($50,000) and a car ($4,000). Offset against those were the following obligations:

Educational loans	$25,000
Life insurance loan	10,000
Professional and personal loans	30,000
Home loan	50,000
Auto loan	4,000
Total	$119,000

Up to this point, the doctor and his wife had been fairly conservative. However, as they began to feel the full impact of monthly loan payments, living expenses, and practice costs, they reacted. Without advice from an attorney or accountant, he began to build up office payables, and they began to run up credit card charges and charge accounts with local merchants. They further overcommitted themselves by purchasing an $85,000 house and buying new office equipment. By now, their total indebtedness had swelled to well above $150,000. At this point, one bad investment was all that was needed to cause the American dream to end in personal bankruptcy. Sadly, this young medical couple's experience with personal bankruptcy is not uncommon.

Although physicians earn a great deal of money—despite extensive losses from operating inefficient offices and payment of high rates of income tax—medical accountants and attorneys report that probably no more than 10 to 20 percent of physician families save on a systematic basis to build a cash reserve. The majority live beyond their means by adopting a standard of living that commits every dollar of income. Although they may have some assets, they have little or no cash reserve. Sometimes the cause is the physician's wife and family, who may desire expensive country club memberships, large homes in affluent neighborhoods, cars, and travel, and thus present the breadwinner with an insoluble financial problem. Or the physician himself may prompt the spending. In either instance, overspending is a way of life for a large majority of physician families. The problem affects all ages. Middle-aged physicians worry as much about meeting college tuition costs as do young physicians about meeting home mortgage payments. Once overextended, the physician's only recourse is to work harder in an attempt to generate more revenue.

Medical accountants and attorneys also estimate that at any point in time 10 to 20 percent of physicians are in serious financial trouble. Persons in this group are typically those who cannot resist the pressures to live beyond their means. The case of "Dr. Charles Dudley Warner" in Chapter Two is an example of this problem. His earnings might well cover the cost of his expensive home. But his home, the private clubs, the private colleges for his children, the expensive office setting, all have contributed to his present desperate condition. "Dr. Warner" has long since given up hope of accumulating a retirement fund sufficient to support him and his wife in their accustomed fashion. This situation might seem improbable for a man who doubtlessly advises others on the importance of protecting their health in the future. But the judgment of those who are intimately familiar with the financial planning habits of large numbers of physicians is that only a minority of physicians adequately prepare for retirement or poor health. Their estimate is that, at retirement age, about 50 percent of physicians own only their homes, some meager savings, and their practices. Physicians' estates are amazingly small when compared with the large incomes they generated during their working lives.

Often the physician in financial trouble makes the most pessimistic assessment of his ability to improve his situation. He may reason that of his $100,000 gross revenue last year, about half remained as taxable income after paying his office expenses. Taxes took 30 percent of that, so that he netted about $35,000 for himself and his family. Faced with the reality that his family is already committed to spending $45,000 per year, he may reason that his only recourse is to increase his gross revenue by $30,000 (three times the $10,000 shortfall). Thus, he would need a gross revenue of $130,000 rather than the $100,000 he is currently earning. Compound this problem, then, with a $10,000 increase in malpractice insurance rates and the physician will panic. He sees no way that his medical business can tolerate such rapid increases in overhead, especially at a time when he is struggling to cope with the increasing costs of his personal life and with inflationary pressures as well. Seldom does it occur to him that a combination of reduced spending and improved office efficiency could bring him financial solvency without the work required to generate $30,000 additional gross revenue.

In such instances, the physician's financial situation could be improved considerably if he would seek the advice of a competent lawyer, accountant, or business consultant. Such professionals could help him and his family set up a financial plan to pay off their debts and reduce their spending. They could also help him improve the efficiency of his practice. But too often the physician would interpret the inevitable demand for moderation in spending as sermonizing. Few financial advisors can recall when such advice was heeded by medical families.

The physician seldom presents his financial problems to a lawyer, accountant, or business consultant. They may cost the physician more than he thinks he can afford. Most physicians seek the help of an attorney only when they want to make a will, obtain a divorce, or form a corporation for tax sheltering purposes. Similarly, they approach their accountants for little else than preparing the financial statements required to calculate income taxes. Thus, the physician will use neither lawyers nor accountants for financial advice—business or personal—until his situation becomes desperate. Ironically, a profession as highly specialized as medicine is made up of practitioners who are unwilling to employ the services of specialists in other professions. If the physician consults with anyone concerning business, he usually does so with another doctor. But, with their common lack of business acumen, they are of little help to each other.

Divorce is becoming increasingly common in medical families. According to interviews with attorneys and accountants, money problems figure prominently in the breakup of many medical marriages. But the financial cost of divorce is especially severe for the physician. His wife has become accustomed to his earnings and most likely has developed tastes and spending habits that are not easily reversed. She typically does not work, and few courts would expect her to begin working in middle age, particularly if she stood by her husband through the lean years of medical training and establishing his practice. Surprised at the paucity of assets in most medical families, the wife's attorney usually designates the physician's practice as the principal family asset and appeals to the court to award her a settlement for her part-ownership in the medical practice developed during the years of their marriage. The result usually is a divorce settlement that extracts payment to the wife for her share of the medical practice, and the physician must honor this obligation if he is to retain ownership of his only means of support. He will then use that practice to generate the revenues necessary to provide her alimony and child support. Because physicians are responsible people, they commonly continue to give their families a large share of their earnings long after the end of their marriages.

Business Investment

The lack of business acumen of most physicians also contributes to their frequent failure in business investments. Although few means are available to document their poor investment performance, numerous interviews with accountants and attorneys lead to the conclusion that most physicians are exceptionally poor at making investments and that many are easy prey for promoters of ill-advised, and sometimes ludicrous, investment schemes. Stories of personal bankruptcies abound. An article in the *New York Times* is typical of the stories told repeatedly by lawyers and accountants:

> Their naivete makes doctors notoriously easy marks for unscrupulous lawyers and businessmen trying to promote a sharp deal. A Los Angeles legal secretary who asked not to be identified and who has spent some time working for two such attorneys, reports, "The law partners' main preoccupation was dreaming up phony corporations and thinking up schemes to get doctors to invest in them. None of these corporations ever succeeded, but the doctors were suckers and eager to invest. Their contribution ranged from $2,000 to $25,000 and $50,000 each. Doctors who complained about not getting a return on their investment were quickly bought out. The others just dangled. Doctors understand that all patients do not live after surgery, and they seem to take a similar view when a company in which they've invested fails. They are without a doubt the most vulnerable group of investors in the world."
>
> The legal secretary explains the vulnerability of doctors not merely in terms of their lack of business experience; she also suspects that many are tired of merely being doctors and want to swing a little. "Sometimes the riskier or crazier the venture, the more appeal it seems to have for them," she says.
>
> And, indeed, one finds doctors investing in feed-lot cattle, professional baseball and football teams, experimental motion pictures, and exotic resorts. *Medical Economics* frequently runs homiletic stories written by doctors explaining how they have just lost their shirts on some scheme. One article, entitled "Never Invest in Anything that Eats—Like a Horse," describes a group of doctors' brief and unprofitable fling with owning four harness-racing horses. Two other articles—this time written by the editors of *Medical Economics*—describe, first in glowing terms, the nineteen-sixties investments that a group of Chicago doctors were making in Virgin Islands vacation villas ("We invest where we can enjoy it"), and then, in 1974, the bankruptcy of the group owing to overly rapid expansion, plus the decline in tourism after a series of racial murders in St. Croix.[2]

A recent example of the inability of many physicians to evaluate investment opportunities is worth recounting. In 1971, five well-established physicians in a major metropolitan area decided to invest in the development of a training school for health professionals. The school was licensed and staffed to train medical assistants and licensed vocational nurses for employment in physicians' offices. The physician investors saw an opportunity for a profitable investment. Unlike other physicians who agree to unwise investment schemes, these men were confident that they were entering a business that their medical backgrounds would help them to understand and operate. Yet, so sure were they that the school would be an immediate success, they did not retain the services of accountants and attorneys to establish the necessary corporate documents. One important oversight was their failure to apply to the Internal Revenue Service for Subchapter S status that would have allowed each of the investors to take advantage of a tax writeoff for the business losses incurred during the period the school was being established. Furthermore, lack of market analysis and poor management soon created the need for large sums of additional money. These funds were raised by the gradual sale of stock to a total of twenty-four investors, five of whom were patients of the original physician investors. The total cash investment made by a physician was $30,000; the largest investment made by a patient was $20,000.

Realizing that they needed management help, the group hired an experienced businessman to head the school. This man also lent $68,000 to the school. Under his leadership, however, it continued to lose money. Even so, the group allowed him to take a majority equity interest in order to retain his participation. At this critical time, additional sums that were lent to the school by nine physicians and patient investors, together with the director's loan of $68,000, brought the total to $378,000.

The school continued to lose money, and eventually the investment group required a large bank loan to remain open. Not all shareholders in the company agreed to guarantee the loan. Ten investors guaranteed $99,000 in loans, only $30,000 of which gave further stock participation to four of those ten participants. The remaining $69,000 in guarantees was provided by the investors without stock reimbursement. When faced with pressure from the bank for repayment of principal and interest, three of the physicians gave still more money amounting to $16,000.

In the end, the school for health professionals went bankrupt, despite the doctors' hope that their understanding of this type of business would ensure its success. Unfortunately, the doctors did not know that schools of this type were increasing in number and were having difficulty placing their students. The result was a decline in student demand for schools with this training capability. The total losses of the twenty-four investors over a period of three years exceeded $600,000. This experience did not end, however, with these massive personal losses. Six of the investors were held responsible for more than $50,000 in unpaid withholding taxes because of their willingness to assume personal obligations not accepted by all the shareholders in unison. One of the physicians who had been most active in the solicitation of this investment opportunity with his patients is being sued for $25,000 in invested capital and faces charges of fraud. He and at least one other participating physician are considering declaring personal bankruptcy to protect themselves from the prospect of complete financial disaster for themselves and their families.

In their ability to earn large sums of money without business training or business acumen, physicians resemble professional athletes and entertainers more than they do businessmen. On occasion, one hears of bad investments made by architects, engineers, and attorneys, to be sure. But typically, people in most businesses and professions, to have accumulated funds for investment, will necessarily have developed a business background. Physicians, by contrast, like athletes and entertainers, are exceptions. And like the quarterback and the actor, they often overspend and make bad investments, most of which are ill conceived and some of which are fraudulent. Nonetheless, physicians seldom find the time and are usually disinclined to make the effort to learn how to invest wisely. Such a learning process takes years of study and experience and an ability that is selectively developed by the successful members of other professions.

SOME STRATEGIC BUSINESS DECISIONS

The most crucial business decisions in managing a medical practice, as in any business, are those infrequently made strategic choices about the nature of the practice. How many physicians should be included in the practice? How many aides should be hired, and what kinds of aides should they be? Should the practice buy certain specialized equipment, and when is it better to send patients to outside facilities such as laboratories and radiology centers for diagnostic work or therapy?

No one in medical school taught the physician how to analyze these questions. He is not likely to want to seek the advice of consultants, except perhaps to talk with some other physicians who probably know little more about the subject than he does. Should he prove to be the exception who does seek such advice, he will have great difficulty in knowing when he has found a competent adviser.

Although many management consultants will be eager to help him set up his practice, they can be expensive, are sometimes dishonest, and too often are not qualified to help with the fundamental strategic questions involved in organizing a medical practice.

Most of the physicians' strategic decisions are made with only the most meager information. Some talk to a few people and then make a decision—often an impulsive one. They borrow money, form partnerships, sign contracts for office space and equipment, and hire personnel, frequently with only a dim awareness of available alternatives and the possible outcome of the choices they make.

Some critics of the health care system have suggested that the strategic business decisions now being made by physicians are not optimal from a social perspective. They argue that medical care could be delivered for less cost by increased use of physician aides, expanded deployment of medical equipment, and group practice.

Is it true that expanded use of physician aides, greater use of medical equipment, and group practice have the potential to increase the productivity of medical practice in the United States? The typical physician is not likely to know the answer to this question, nor how to go about finding it. Yet, in thousands of medical practices across the country, physicians are making decisions that have the effect of being strategic for the working of the health care delivery system.

A fairly substantial body of knowledge is available to help in assessing the opportunities for increasing the efficiency of medical practice. Chapters Four to Six in Part III will examine this evidence.

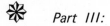 *Part III:*

Opportunities for Increasing the Efficiency of Medical Practice

Chapter Four

The Use of Medical Aides

The most costly and important resource in the medical office is the physician's time. Given this obvious fact, what is the most efficient way for the physician to organize his office? In particular, to what extent could the typical medical practice efficiently and profitably use more aides without jeopardizing the quality of the care that it delivers? Decisions on the use of medical aides must be based on the following factors:

The kinds of tasks performed in the medical practice;
The tasks that could be delegated to aides without reducing the quality of care;
The relationship between the number of aides employed and the physician's productivity;
The acceptability of medical aides to physicians and their patients.

An authority on this subject is Uwe Reinhardt of Princeton University. He has classified the tasks performed in medical offices as clerical, information gathering, diagnostic, and therapeutic.[1] The clerical category includes such tasks as making appointments, filing and retrieving patient records, filling out insurance forms, billing patients and receiving payments, and doing routine bookkeeping. Although the physician is capable of performing these tasks himself, his time would not be used to the best advantage in this work and many, if not all, of these jobs can be delegated to nonphysicians with no loss whatsoever in the quality of patient care.

Information gathering consists of collecting information from patients through taking patient histories or conducting physical examinations. Some of these tasks can be delegated by the physician (drawing a blood sample) while others cannot (examining the retina of the eye). The extent to which physicians delegate data-gathering tasks to aides varies widely from physician to physician, as will be demonstrated.

The diagnostic category consists of interpreting the information collected in the data-gathering stage. Diagnosis may take the form of drawing inferences from information acquired in a physical examination and may include interpreting results of x-rays or laboratory tests. The delegation of work to aides is less desirable in diagnosis than in the other three task categories, but even in diagnosis some degree of delegation is possible. For example, when a patient calls the office with a complaint, an aide may listen to a description of the symptoms and decide whether or not the physician should be consulted. The extent to which aides are permitted to perform diagnostic tasks also varies fairly widely in medical practice.

The therapeutic category includes administering medicine; giving immunizations; suturing or dressing wounds; counselling patients about diets, exercise, smoking, or drug regimens; providing therapy of many kinds (e.g., inhalation therapy, physical therapy, psychological therapy, radiation therapy, and chemotherapy); and surgery. Again, the degree to which these tasks are delegated differs greatly from one medical practice to another. In many practices, a large number of these tasks are delegated to aides; in recent years, many new physician assistant roles have been created to provide manpower for physicians who wish to delegate therapeutic tasks.

To explore the subject further, Reinhardt has classified the full set of tasks that could be delegated:

Type I. Those tasks that will always be prescribed by the physician but that will be produced on his premises only if he has the appropriate staff, failing which they will be produced by outside facilities.

Type II. Those tasks the physician prescribes only if he employs sufficient staff to perform them, failing which they will not be performed at all in the management of the condition.

Type III. Those tasks that will always be prescribed by the physician and performed in his practice either by him (in the absence of support personnel) or by him and any staff he employs.[2]

Reinhardt notes that the hiring of aides to perform Type I tasks does not increase the physician's productivity, although it may enlarge the gross receipts of his practice and increase his profits. If the additional personnel require that the physician spend more time supervising them, they might actually decrease his productivity. From an overall perspective, however, bringing new service capability into the medical practice has the potential to reduce total patient cost by combining several medical tasks during a single visit.

If an increase in the number of aides merely increases the output of Type II services, two possibilities might be realized. One is that some of these services may not be necessary from a strictly medical perspective. The other is that the added services may improve the quality of care given in the practice.

Using aides to perform Type III tasks offers the greatest potential for increasing physician productivity. Regarding the delegation of such tasks, Reinhardt concludes:

> Careful task analysis of medical practices with a variety of staffing patterns, and in a variety of medical specialties, has indicated that far too many physicians still routinely perform tasks that could just as safely be performed by intermediate- and lower-level health workers or by clerical personnel. There is also evidence that where intermediate-level health workers are employed, they are usually burdened with tasks that should really be delegated to lower-level assistants. In other words, neither physicians nor physician extenders seem to be used to maximum effectiveness.[3]

In support of his conclusion, Reinhardt cites a study of pediatrics by Alfred Yankauer and his associates that makes it clear that physicians vary a great deal in the extent to which they are willing to delegate tasks to aides. These authors presented the data shown in Table 4-1 on delegation of medical tasks. These findings not only support Reinhardt's conclusion but also demonstrate a strong association between task delegation and the number of aides employed by each physician.

Many other studies have also claimed that physician productivity and earnings could be increased if more tasks were delegated to aides. Table 4-2 reports typical results. Even though the average physician employs only slightly more than two aides, these findings show that aides contribute substantially to practice productivity up to four aides or more. A study of solo general practitioners summarized in Table 4-3 further demonstrates this point.

It should be pointed out that the evidence presented so far concerns only the technical feasibility of utilizing aides to increase physician productivity. Of more significance is the question of economic feasibility—that is, how many aides ought a physician to hire, taking into account both the increases in output and increases in costs that would occur if aide utilization increased?

Table 4-1. Percentage of Times Selected Tasks Were Performed by Pediatricians

	Total Number of Health Workers Employed				
	1-1.5	*2-2.5*	*3-3.5*	*4-4.5*	*5 or more*
Technical Tasks					
Weighing	32	9	8	1	2
Body Measurements	46	19	17	13	10
Immunizations	75	42	35	27	18
Parenteral Drugs	81	50	41	32	25
Vision Screening	44	24	16	13	8
Hearing Screening	54	44	39	34	22
Developmental Screening	73	70	69	61	65
Laboratory Tasks					
Hemoglobin/Hematocrit	44	22	18	13	4
Urinalysis	38	36	18	16	7
Blood Count/Smear	21	17	15	9	4
Clerical Tasks					
Inventory/Supply	11	3	3	2	2
Growth Charting	49	42	42	51	44
Insurance Forms	22	10	8	8	6

Source: A. Yankauer, J. P. Connelly, and J. J. Feldman, "Task Performance and Task Delegation in Pediatric Office Practice," *American Journal of Public Health,* vol. 59 (July 1969), p. 1108. Cited in Reinhardt, *Physician Productivity and the Demand for Health Manpower, An Economic Analysis* (Cambridge, Mass: Ballinger Publishing Company, 1975), p. 112.

Table 4-2. Apparent Effect of Auxiliary Personnel and the Number of Examination Rooms on Physician Productivity

Number of Examining Rooms per Solo M.D.	Number of Full-Time Office Aides	Physician's Total Professional Hours per Week	Office Visits per Week	Practice Gross	Practice Net
5 or more	3	66	164	$96,200	$51,380
4	2	63	154	79,810	44,460
3	2	63	115	64,610	37,470
2	1	62	87	58,500	35,900
1	0	58	45	45,800	32,560

Source: A. Owens, "How Many Doctors are Really Working at Full Capacity?" *Medical Economics* (January 18, 1971), p. 93. Cited in Reinhardt, *Physician Productivity and the Demand for Health Manpower,* p. 114.

Reinhardt discovered that:

The average practice in our sample could have *profitably* employed close to four aides per physician or twice the observed sample average. Had the

Table 4-3. Estimated Effect of Physician Hours and of Aides on the Rate of Physician Output (Solo General Practitioners)

Number of Physician Hours per Week	Number of Aides per Physician						
	0	.5	1	2	3	4	5
Total Practice Hours	Total Patient Visits Per Week						
40	85	96	107	128	146	159	165
60	123	139	155	185	212	230	239
Office Hours	Office Visits Per Week						
25	73	85	99	122	142	154	156
35	91	107	122	153	178	193	196
Total Practice Hours	Patient Billings Per Year						
40	28.1	32.1	36.1	43.9	50.8	55.7	58.1
60	36.0	41.1	46.2	56.3	65.0	71.4	74.4

* In thousands of dollars, based on 1965 income data.
Source: U.E. Reinhardt, "A Production Function for Physician Services," *Review of Economics and Statistics*, vol. 54, no. 1 (February 1972), p. 63.

physicians actually employed this higher number of aides, then their weekly number of total patient visits would have been about 25 percent higher than the current average of 183, while their weekly number of *office* visits would have been about 28 percent higher than the current average of 151 visits.[4]

Reinhardt has estimated that a 4 percent increase in physician productivity would be equivalent to society's gaining the care of the entire graduating classes of all the medical schools in the United States. His estimate suggests, then, that by efficiently employing aides, physicians might generate productivity increases equivalent to the total output of new physicians of all medical schools for a period of six or seven years.

Using different data and methodology, Larry Kimbell and Robert Deane at the University of Southern California also estimated that physicians could profitably hire three to four aides and in doing so could increase their gross billings by about 12 percent, or the equivalent of 16.9 million annual patient visits per year.[5]

Both the Reinhardt and the Kimbell and Deane study define aides to include all nurses, clerical workers, and technicians. The great majority of such aides in small-scale private practice are clerical workers and nurses. Advocates of the concept of increasing physician productivity through the use of physician assistants, however, envisage making much greater use of them than is now common. Dr. William Schwartz, chief of medicine at Tufts New England Medical Center, believes:

... there seems little question that physicians' assistants, taking patient histories, carrying out physical examinations, and administering intravenous fluids, can greatly augment the efficiency of the doctor. . . . I would like to suggest, however, that this approach to the use of non-physicians is much too limited. It is conceivable that by going further we can produce a revolution in the use of health manpower in which the physician's efforts are truly reserved for those tasks which require his high level of skill, education and intellect. I am suggesting, in other words, that if we undertake a rigorous analysis of what the doctor does, we will almost certainly find that a substantial number of his tasks, now considered sacrosanct, could be done instead by skilled technicians who could be quickly trained for single specialized tasks: for example, to diagnose and treat simple fractures, remove an appendix, strip varicose veins, carry out therapeutic abortions, or perform needle biopsies of the kidney and liver. Such new uses of manpower could well free a significant additional fraction of the physician's time.[6]

If physician assistants were ever to be used that extensively, the increases in health care productivity would be enormous. Research by Richard Zeckhauser and Michael Eliastam at Harvard University indicated that ". . . when taking on his most productive assignments, it is found, a physician assistant can replace half of a full-time doctor."[7]

A number of universities are now training people to perform tasks traditionally reserved for physicians. For example, the University of California at Los Angeles has a program to train nurse-midwives. These assistants can give cancer tests, follow pregnancies, deliver babies, and provide postpartum care. A study of patient acceptance of these physician aides revealed that many female patients preferred to receive such services as the insertion of intrauterine devices by paramedical personnel rather than from the obstetrician-gynecologist.[8]

The University of Washington has an ambitious program to train former military corpsmen for civilian service in medical offices. They are trained to give physical examinations, prescribe commonly used medications, provide health education counselling, and perform some minor surgery. They are placed in medical offices in isolated or disadvantaged areas of the Northwest. Available evidence indicates that they are well received by most patients.[9]

Despite the favorable outcome of many physician aide programs, the concept of using medical assistants as physician extenders—that is, as substitutes for physicians in diagnosis and therapy—is meeting with a great deal of resistance from doctors. Physicians worry that the use of extenders will reduce the quality of their care. They also fear that permitting extenders to diagnose and treat patients will increase their chances of becoming involved in costly malpractice suits. Finally, boards of medical examiners in most states have been slow to authorize the use of extenders. For all of these reasons, in all likelihood the use of physician extenders will never become widespread in fee-for-service, office-based medical practice.

In the prepaid group setting, however, extenders are used quite successfully. Kaiser employs them with good effect; patients have learned through experience that extenders are competent and fully acceptable in performing their assigned tasks. Kaiser, with its managerial sophistication, is less likely to be concerned about malpractice suits resulting from the use of extenders. Its size permits it to self-insure against malpractice claims.

Physicians in office-based practices, however, need not go so far as to use full physician extenders to increase the productivity of their practices. Instead, aides can be employed to perform numerous routine tasks, such as administering tests for vision and hearing, taking electrocardiograms and x-rays, weighing infants, giving shots, and even eliciting much of the patient's medical history. Physicians throughout the country are now doing many of these simple tasks themselves.

To summarize, available evidence suggests that potential increases in the productivity of medical practice by means of physician extenders and assistants are quite substantial. This evidence indicates that hiring more assistants to perform routine tasks might increase the productivity of the physician's time by 10 to 25 percent,[10] and the employment of full physician extenders can increase a physician's ability to see patients by 50 percent.[11]

But most office-based physicians see no reason to increase the size of their staffs. Some fear that increasing their staff will raise their overhead and thus reduce their incomes. Others can muster little enthusiasm for office management; they do not like to plan, organize, and direct the work of others. Moreover, most physicians are too unskilled in management to be able to see ways to make productive use of aides. So long as small-scale, fee-for-service medical practice is the norm in the United States, little improvement in medical productivity based on the improved use of aides can be expected.

※ *Chapter Five*

Technology in Medicine

Medical technology has advanced enormously in recent decades and has led to many innovations that have radically altered hospital and some private office medical care. Two kinds of questions can be asked about these technical advances. First, do they contribute meaningfully to the quality of care, and, second, do they improve the efficiency of tasks performed by the physician and by other members of the physician's team as well?

Two types of equipment technology should be distinguished. The first is equipment used to help the physician in the practice of medicine. The other is used to assist him and his staff in performing such tasks as billing and records keeping.

New machines to help care for patients have proved to be a mixed blessing to medicine. On the one hand, new technology increases the capability of physicians to diagnose and treat medical problems; on the other, it adds to the complexity and cost of medicine. Two examples will illustrate this point.

Stress electrocardiography is a medical test performed by having a patient exercise to a measured degree of effort while the electrocardiogram is being monitored. In the 1960s, the patient was tested while walking up and down a two-step block until his pulse rate reached a critical value or until he had exercised for a prescribed period of time. The patient was charged approximately $50 for the test. The drawback was that no effective measure of the amount of work done by the patient was possible. Consequently, the procedure was changed to one in which the patient rode a stationary bicycle against a known amount of resistance. The bicycle cost $1,000 and the patient was charged about $75. Physicians subsequently recognized that walking up and down a step or riding on a bicycle are not common forms of exertion. Consequently, the test has been improved so that now the patient walks on a treadmill. As the test progresses, the speed of the treadmill and its incline are gradually increased. Given a patient's age and sex, the maximum pulse rate at which the patient is expected to become totally exhausted can be predicted. The patient is taken to 90 percent of that maximum pulse rate, if possible.

With the traditional resting electrocardiogram, which is taken with the patient lying down, about 5 percent of the population shows some abnormal signs. But with the stress electrocardiogram done on a treadmill, abnormalities are recorded in about one-third of the population. Thus, the internist has strong evidence that he can improve the quality of his cardiac evaluations if he has the capability to perform stress electrocardiography in his office. But a multiple channel stress electrocardiogram machine costs about $6,000. Another $3,000 must be spent for the treadmill, bringing the total to $9,000. In addition to the cost of the equipment, the physician must allocate space for it and provide a shower for patients to use after the test is completed. Furthermore, he must spend an additional $1,000 for a defibrillator in anticipation of cardiac emergencies that might be precipitated by the test. He must hire a nurse trained to perform electrocardiograms or hire a skilled ECG technician. He must also train his staff in cardiopulmonary resuscitation. Once he has made all of these investments and begins to perform stress electrocardiography in his office, the physician must make himself available throughout each test so that he can observe continuous test results as the test is performed. All of this naturally adds to practice costs.

Before stress electrocardiography, when electrocardiograms were done with the patient at rest, the test cost about $30; with a treadmill it costs the patient approximately $100. Thus, a technological advance has improved the quality of care, but it has also added to the complexity of the medical practice. The possibility of a mishap in the physician's office has also increased greatly. And the capacity to perform stress electrocardiography in the physician's office certainly does not save his time. To date, not many physicians have acquired the capability to do stress electrocardiography in their offices, but most internists are feeling some pressure to do so.

A logical question, perhaps, is why medical entrepreneurs do not establish businesses that specialize in stress electrocardiography? The answer is that a number have been started and have been unsuccessful. One physician provided such a service, and at the end of a year's operation had received only three referrals from the physicians in his area. Physicians may be reluctant to refer their patients to a setting that is obviously technically more sophisticated than their own. Moreover, by referring his patients to another source of care, the physician also forfeits income.

A second example of the way that technology adds to the complexity and cost of medicine is the computer-assisted tomographic scanner, initially marketed in 1972 by EMI, a large British electronics company. The EMI device can take a scanning x-ray of different levels of the brain and simultaneously compare it with the normal brain by computer analysis. Abnormal findings such as tumors or hemorrhage are then displayed by the computer on a television screen or recorded in a computer printout.

The EMI brain scanners cost about $500,000. Because of their slow operation, each of these scanners is capable of handling only ten to twelve patient cases per day. Utilization of a scanner by a hospital or large clinic also requires a radiologist with special training in neuroradiology to be responsible for interpretations. As soon as the EMI brain scanner became available, virtually every academic medical center and major medical clinic in America purchased one. Yet, there was evidence that EMI would have a total body scanner available within two years, which would make obsolete the specialized brain scanner. Another well-known fact was that U.S. companies such as General Electric, Pfizer, Varian Associates and Ohio-Nuclear were considering developing or already had prototypes of competitive brain scanners. In fact, within two years after the EMI brain scanner appeared on the market, both EMI and a U.S. company offered a total body scanner. The price of the total body scanners may vary from $500,000 to $1 million.

So while revolutionary developments were taking place in the development of scanners, medical schools and prestigious medical clinics began to purchase brain scanners. The hospitals and large clinics were next to join the rush for scanners. Their eagerness to purchase brain scanners appears to have been motivated mainly by their desire to maintain or enhance the reputation of their institutions. Some hospitals also wished to buy scanners because they anticipated that government regulations might later limit the purchase of such equipment. The needs of patients and the community appear to have been less important considerations.

The original brain scanners operate so slowly that their owners have had to charge as much as $250 for a single test. Should new, faster scanners be developed—and such scanners are being brought into the market—then tests could be offered for significantly less money. But what hospital staff wanted to wait for the improved scanners before purchasing one?

So many hospitals and clinics have purchased scanners that few of these machines can be expected to pay for themselves if they are used only for the purpose they were intended—that is, for diagnosis of suspected brain tumors or intracranial hemorrhages. Clearly, a policy that would have better served the health care consumer and society as a whole would have been to utilize the scanners to serve entire geographic regions in selected hospitals. This approach has been the policy in England, a country that has only five scanners for the entire nation of roughly 50 million people. In the United States, with a population of slightly more than 200 million, approximately 5,000 scanners are in place or have been ordered. American hospitals and clinics cannot resist the urge to have the latest technological innovations, and the government's Comprehensive Health Planning Councils are powerless to do more than recommend to hospitals that they coordinate their equipment purchases.

At present, hospitals, many of which made down payments of $100,000 per machine, are now facing up to a year's wait for delivery of their already outdated brain scanners. Those that have received their scanners report that they are experiencing major difficulties keeping them operating properly. But the rush to acquire them goes on, and it will be followed by a push to acquire total body scanners as soon as they are available.

What happens to the health care consumer during this pursuit of medical technology? Once a brain scanner is put into operation, physicians will want to utilize it. But few cases of potential brain tumor or intracranial hemorrhage occur in a day at a typical hospital. Consequently, to make the most of the capital equipment investment, physicians are beginning to use brain scanners to evaluate that most common of complaints, the headache. The result is that hospitals find justifying purchasing brain scanners is easy, because their staff physicians are anxious to reassure patients that their headaches are not of serious consequence.

Undoubtedly, brain scanners have real medical value, but whether widespread use of them on patients who are suffering from headaches is wise in view of their cost is debatable. One thing is certain, the brain scanner, and the body scanner to follow, have not saved any of the physician's scarce time or increased his productivity.

The community at large will pay for these new scanners through higher health insurance premiums. Medicare, Medicaid, Blue Cross, and private insurance, all of which authorized payment for brain scans, now find themselves inundated with bills for expensive scanning procedures to evaluate minor complaints.

Both stress electrocardiography and tomographic scanners are typical of almost all technological innovations in medicine. They advance the state of the art and provide real medical benefits for some patients. Consequently, physicians are eager to utilize these and other new types of medical equipment. But new technology is frequently expensive and also difficult to evaluate from a social perspective. The costs are apparent and easy to measure, but the benefits—better health for some people for a time—are much more difficult to assess and evaluate. Whether such benefits exceed costs is difficult to determine. Even so, the new technology is invariably adopted because physicians in hospitals, in clinics, and in medical offices want to be able to practice the very best medicine possible, regardless of cost. Most technological innovations also complicate the practice of medicine. New technology seldom makes doctors more productive by serving as a substitute for their time; rather, it requires more of their time.

Perhaps there are exceptions. Claims are made that some equipment may turn out to save physician time. William B. Schwartz has experimented with the use of computers and suggests:

> It seems possible that in the not too distant future the physician and the computer will engage in frequent dialogue, the computer continuously taking note of history, physical findings, laboratory data, and the like, alerting the physician to the most probable diagnoses and suggesting the appropriate, safest course of action. One may thus project a revolution in the health care system in which the importance of remembering facts is sharply reduced, the decision-making process is aided and abetted by computers, and many tasks formerly in the domain of the physician are taken over by a consortium of computers and paramedical personnel.[1]

Other technological advances that are expected to conserve physician time and increase productivity are: picture-phones, telemetry, and two-way television for monitoring distant hospital patients and diagnosing problems of rural patients who may then receive care by physician assistants. However, Reinhardt has cautioned:

> ...for the most part, the availability of [modern equipment for patient care] permits physicians to perform otherwise impossible procedures, to restore health in otherwise untreatable cases, and to maintain life in otherwise hopeless cases.... [T]he availability of this wider range of services

unquestionably enhances the physician's contribution to the health-production process. But the introduction of sophisticated medical equipment also tends to increase the demand for physician services.

. . . if one can judge from past experience in this area, a realistic prognosis seems to be that any future health manpower savings achieved through [substituting machines for physicians and other health workers] is likely to be offset—and perhaps even more than offset—by increases in the demand for health care [brought about by the use of machines themselves], and hence in the demand for all types of health manpower. Such an outcome obviously does not make greater [substitution of machines for physicians] in health care production an unattractive proposition. One merely should not expect the infusion of [machines for patient care] into the health care sector to permit reductions in the aggregate physician-population in future years.[2]

As indicated earlier, a second category of equipment is designed to support the nonmedical work required in medical practice. In the office setting, the two largest applications for such equipment are for records storage and retrieval and for patient billing and accounting.

Accumulating and maintaining medical records is a difficult and costly task in all medical practices. The physician's written and verbally dictated records of patient care must be accurately transcribed by his clerical staff. But dictating into a tape recorder is time-consuming for the physician. Most physicians will readily admit that this aspect of their work is the one that they most dislike. Commonly staff physicians are disciplined by their hospitals for not complying with rules for submitting timely medical record entries; sometimes they are even suspended from the hospital staff for this offense. Hospitals continually have problems with physicians who know that they are being monitored and still do not do an adequate job of dictating medical records. In view of hospital problems in this respect, the chaos in many private medical offices can be easily surmised.

Accurate transcription of medical records is time-consuming and expensive. If the physician hires an unskilled, low-salaried secretary, he will have to make frequent corrections in her work; hence, transcribing costs will probably be higher than if he had hired a competent worker who commanded a substantial salary.

The proper maintaining of complete medical records is not only important to the proper functioning of the medical business office, it is a legal requirement as well. When a practice is new, this requirement does not create any particular problems. As the practice matures, however, and as the volume of medical records increases, the physician's need for ready access to orderly, reproducible records becomes a costly burden. A large part of this cost is the floor space required for filing cabinets since medical records are bulky and x-ray film is physically heavy.

A number of alternatives are available for storing and retrieving records. Some clinics have found, for example, that the cost of microfilming medical records is less than the cost of floor space for storing them. X-rays can also be microfilmed. Despite the advantages of microfilming, however, physicians are reluctant to use this technology. Some fear that the company doing the microfilming will lose part of a patient record—just the page that might be needed to defend against a malpractice suit. Others fear that the quality of reproduction of x-rays will not be adequate to support their interpretation of the original film. Consequently, most physicians prefer to maintain all records in their original form. So with each passing year, the back room becomes jammed with more and more records.

Paperwork is one of the most pressing problems of medical practice, with billing being the most serious. All health care insurance underwriters, including the union-supported health plans, have a different billing form that must be completed by the physician's office staff. Every reporting and billing form for every government health program is different and has a different set of guidelines for usage. Every insurance company requires its own form to report physical examinations, and, parenthetically, a different urine specimen bottle for mailing into the home office. Similarly, all the forms for reporting injuries for insurance companies, trade union benefit programs, and state and federal agencies are different. The director of one clinic reports that individual patients have given him as many as twelve different forms to fill out in a one-month period. An overworked internist in solo practice, pointing to a pile of paperwork that had backed up from his secretary's desk to his own, noted in disgust: "If anyone wants to know why it is impossible to earn a living practicing medicine any more, there is the answer."

Numerous companies have sprung up to offer the physician complete business office systems. But so far they have found physicians to be a most elusive market. The smaller companies do not last very long. For a number of years, such major companies as Technicon, Northrop, Control Data, and IBM have tried to penetrate this potential market, but with little success.

One reason physicians are slow to invest in automated office management systems is that many of them have had very poor experience with companies providing computer billing services. One physician in Los Angeles lost three months of billing records at a company that was processing them when the sheriff's department put a padlock on the company's door as it went into bankruptcy. But quality billing services are available. A number of commercial banks will process billings, handle payrolls, and provide the physician, in addition, with reports on such things as his productivity and the aging of his accounts receivable. These services are attractive and reliable, but expensive.

The potential for improving billing and medical records keeping by automation is very great. NASA's Iliac system at Ames Research Center, California, has enough computer memory capability to store every medical record in the United States. But computer systems for records storage have been slow to develop because of the impossible task of getting physician practices, clinics, and hospitals—not to mention unions, government, and health insurance underwriters—to agree to utilize common forms of data input.

Nonetheless, even the common means of making additions to medical records can be easily improved. Instead of using the customary dictation technique found in offices everywhere, physicians can use mark sense cards and carefully designed medical forms for this purpose. All routine information can be indicated by checking an appropriate place on a form, and the physician can limit his dictation to a description of abnormal findings. An orthopedist in Michigan used to spend an hour with each new case, half an hour with the patient and half an hour with a dictating machine. Using mark sense forms, he now spends a half-hour with each new patient and only fifteen to twenty minutes in dictation. Consequently, he has been able to increase his capacity to see new patients from four to five per half-day. An available commercial system would allow the surgeon to spend half an hour with each patient and only ten to fifteen minutes with dictation. This scheduling would increase his productive capability to six new patients per half-day.

Thus, a simple system is available that would increase by 50 percent the capacity of a physician to see new patients (established patients require far less dictation of records than new patients). But, unlike most businessmen, physicians are apparently less than enthusiastic about such cost-saving innovations. Although the simple system described and other more elaborate but cost-effective computer systems have been commercially available for a number of years, they are largely unsold. As eager as physicians are to innovate with new technology when practicing medicine, they are very conservative about adopting new business procedures. Perhaps the physician does not understand these new systems; perhaps he is not interested in trying to improve the business side of his practice. Very probably, he does not feel confident that he has the experience and background needed to adopt a new business system.

Because the market for medical business systems has been so elusive, companies now allocate little money to research, develop, or improve them. The microfiche system of 3M Company and the physicians' billing and accounting systems of IBM have changed very little in more than five years. Lockheed, which developed a sophisticated information system for hospitals, has given up trying to market it and has sold the system to another company.

In summary, new technology for patient care seldom is cost saving, and typically it requires more, not less, of the physician's time. The physician is eager to adopt this kind of innovation. By contrast, innovations that can reduce the cost of paperwork in hospitals and physicians' offices seldom interest the physician. The potential for improved cost effectiveness in utilizing such technology, however, is quite large.

✳ *Chapter Six*

Optimal Scale of the
Medical Practice

A tradition of American medicine has been the belief that a small office setting provides the best combination of economic efficiency and medical quality. Costs are low, allegedly, because unnecessary overhead expenses can be kept to a minimum. Patients who require specialized equipment can be sent to pathology laboratories, treatment centers, and hospitals. In recent years, however, critics of this type of medical practice have argued that medicine is too complicated to be practiced by relatively isolated physicians in a fragmented "cottage industry" setting and that better quality can be provided at a lower price in a larger organization setting—for example, in a large-scale group practice.

Unfortunately, answering the technical question about which size yields the lowest cost per patient is complicated by a number of factors. For one thing, as the number of physicians in a practice increases, the mix of people, equipment, and available services offered by that practice also changes. Quality characteristics of the health care system may also vary with practice size. For example, in a small setting, the emotional concerns of patients may be emphasized more than they are in a large clinic setting, where greater emphasis may be placed on the technological side of medical practice. Since both of these attributes are prized by patients and physicians alike, the extent to which they occur is likely to influence strongly the appraisal of practice size. Thus, when an economist compares the cost per patient visit in practices of different size, he probably is not comparing the cost of a uniform service.

In estimating whether there are "economies of scale"—that is, whether the cost per patient rises, falls, or remains constant with an increase in practice size—the economist must try by statistical means to control variations in the nature of the output being produced and the mix of inputs being employed. Advanced statistical techniques are available for this purpose, but nonetheless the task is difficult.

Economies of scale in production processes result from several factors. Reinhardt provides an appropriate summary of how these factors may lead to economies of scale in medicine:

> First, some inputs into the production process—for example, x-ray machines or autoclaves—are indivisible in the sense that they are highly specialized and can be used to capacity only for very large patient loads. Second, increases in the scale of production make possible ever finer division of tasks among inputs and thus permit specialization among even those inputs—paramedical personnel and primary care physicians for example—that are not inherently specialized to perform only one or a narrow range of tasks. Such specialization increases the productivity of the inputs involved. Third, the precision with which the daily mix of cases coming to a medical practice can be predicted is apt to increase with the average daily rate of patient flow. Greater accuracy in this prediction, in turn, tends to permit superior scheduling of all types of health personnel and may thus increase manpower productivity. Finally, large-scale production runs usually permit bulk purchasing of at least some inputs and thus permit the purchaser to reap scale economies generated elsewhere. Large group practices, for example, have been found to enjoy economies in the procurement of drugs and medical supplies. Such economies, however, have no direct effect on manpower productivity.[1]

In a society where the advantages of large-scale technology in automobile, steel, and chemical production are well understood, this kind of theoretical case can be very convincing. For example, in *The Doctor Shortage*, the economist Rashi Fein argues:

> ... it would, after all, be quite unusual if there were no economies of scale in the provision of physician services. It is difficult to think of any area of activity in which economies of scale are nonexistent. While this observation cannot be considered proof that economies do exist, this writer would conclude that the "burden of proof" should be on those who deny their existence rather than on others to demonstrate that they are present.[2]

The trouble with such an argument, as Reinhardt and a number of other economists have pointed out, is that it ignores another phenomenon—that is, "diseconomies of scale." Some services and products—for example, those offered by gasoline stations, shoe repair stores, and barber shops—are produced most efficiently in the small business setting.

Diseconomies of scale may occur in medicine because, as the practice expands, its physician manager must spread himself thinner and thinner as he tries to control its operation. This situation can lead to inefficiency and rising costs. Conversely, creating a bureaucracy to manage a practice could also lead to an increase in the cost per patient visit. A related factor is that, as a practice grows, its managers will find it increasingly difficult to coordinate its parts—that is, doctors, allied health personnel, medical records, collections, and so forth. Another key managerial problem that arises in group practices is related to incentives. In a profit-sharing group, the larger the practice, the smaller is the incentive of any doctor to work hard to bring revenue into the practice. Each extra dollar that the physician brings into the group must be shared with other doctors, and his share of the extra dollar decreases as the number of doctors with whom he must divide it increases.[3]

Therefore, the answer as to whether the cost per patient visit of a standardized medical service falls, rises, or remains constant cannot be determined by theory alone. Most likely, some forces are at work to reduce costs as practice size increases at the same time that other forces are at work to increase costs. Knowing whether there are economies or diseconomies of scale in medical practice requires knowing which forces dominate. Learning the answer requires a careful examination of empirical evidence.

Approximately a dozen major studies have explored the issue of economies of scale in medical practice. Together, these studies and professional criticism of them lead to three major conclusions.

First, as shown in Table 6-1, group practice, except for the very

Table 6-1. Average Net Income by Type of Practice, Estimated 1974

Type of Practice	Estimated 1974
Total	$51,621
Solo	47,229
2-Man	61,306
3-Man	58,957
4-Man	56,794
5- to 7-Man	61,194
8- to 25-Man	52,360
26-Man and Over	48,821

Source: American Medical Association, J. R. Cantwell, ed., *Profile of Medical Practice, 1975-76* (Chicago: Center for Health Services Research and Development, American Medical Association, 1976), p. 168. Reprinted by permission of the American Medical Association.

largest groups, is more profitable for physicians than is solo practice. · This evidence is sometimes taken as proof that group practice is more efficient than solo practice, at least up to a certain size. Although such evidence certainly explains why physicians might prefer group practice, it does not substantiate the claim that group practice is less costly per patient visit than is solo practice. Richard Bailey of the University of California at Berkeley discovered that the superior income of a sample of internists in group practice could be accounted for by the fact that they were more likely than solo practitioners to provide ancillary services such as x-ray and laboratory tests "in-house" rather than sending the work outside.[4] The internists in Bailey's sample earned higher incomes than the solo practitioners simply because they had entered a new line of business in competition with institutions that provide x-ray and laboratory tests. Superior efficiency of the internists in group practice was not a cause; in fact, the internists in group practice in the Bailey sample actually worked fifteen to thirty hours less per month and saw fewer patients than did the internists in solo practice. Although several other studies have found no support for the Bailey hypothesis, the most careful and comprehensive studies available on the subject of scale economies in medical practice, by Richard Ernst and Herbert Schwartz, do support it.[5]

Second, the statistical evidence on scale economies is consistent with two separate hypotheses. One is that the cost of a standardized unit of care is uniform across all practice sizes. The other is that there are slight economies of scale. In *single specialty groups* these advantages are rapidly exhausted as the practice grows to the size of four to six physicians. For *multispecialty groups* offering comprehensive care, the least-cost size is thirty to fifty-five physicians, although the economies of scale even at that level are not large. A review of several studies indicates the nature of the evidence that supports these two hypotheses.

Joseph Newhouse of the Rand Corporation found that the per patient overhead cost was $4.54 for a sample of private physicians and $14.24 for three clinics.[6] The costs included in the comparison were billing and accounting; medical records keeping; administration of the outpatient departments of the clinics; registration and appointments; clerical, nursing and nonphysician payroll; institutional overhead charged the clinics; and costs of supplies. He used the large differences in overhead cost per patient to support his claim that large practices are more inefficient than small ones because physicians in group practices with profit-sharing arrangements have less incentive to work hard seeing patients as the number of physicians in the group increases.

The fact that one practice has higher overhead expenses than another, however, does not mean that it is less efficient. Overhead includes only the *nonphysician costs* of running a practice. A medical practice in which physicians do their own appointment setting, reception work, bookkeeping, billing, and collecting would have a very low overhead per patient, but this approach would be very inefficient because it would be wasteful of physician time. Indeed, one of the claims made in favor of group practice is that it is efficient because it substitutes nonphysician labor for physician time whenever possible.

A similar error, frequently made, is to compute the ratio of overhead to gross revenue—that is, the nonphysician expenses of a practice divided by the total collections of the practice—and use that as a measure of practice efficiency. If one practice mode has a ratio of 50 percent and another a ratio of 60 percent, analysts who make this error would claim the former is more efficient. For example, these ratios are reported regularly in *Medical Economics*, a magazine about practice management for physicians, and are interpreted as a measure of practice efficiency. But if one follows this logic to the extreme, then the most efficient medical practice would be run by a physician who sees all of his patients by walking to their homes or to the hospital, providing only his own services, and receiving payment in cash at the time services are performed. With such great effort, this physician might be able to keep his overhead at zero. Clearly, though, his practice would not be efficient. A simple numerical example, shown in Table 6-2, illustrates the point that a low ratio

Table 6-2. The Ratio of Overhead to Gross Revenue: A Hypothetical Example

	Physician				
	A	B	C	D	E
Gross Revenue	$15	$50	$100	$145	$200
Expenses	$ 0	$25	$ 60	$ 95	$140
Net Income	$15	$25	$ 40	$ 50	$ 60
Expenses as a Percent of Gross Revenue	0%	50%	60%	65%	70%

of expenses to gross revenue cannot be interpreted as a measure of practice efficiency. Consider five hypothetical physicians, A, B, C, D, and E. In this table, expenses as a percentage of gross revenue rises with the size of the practice, but so does net income. What physician would not choose Practice E? It has an overhead of 70 percent, but its net income of $60,000 per year is the largest of all the practices shown. On the other hand, other hypothetical data could be contrived to show the most profitable practices are those with low expense to gross revenue ratios. By itself, this ratio tells nothing about the efficiency of a medical practice.

Frederick Golladay, Marilyn Manser, and Kenneth Smith conducted a computer study at the University of Wisconsin to determine how the substitution of ancillary personnel for physician time could promote economies of scale in medical practice. They found that economies of scale were possible, at least in theory, but that "the bulk of these economies are exploited by three-physician practices where physician extenders are not allowed to be employed, or by two-physician groups where physician extenders are used."[7] Even under ideal conditions, where the physician is assumed—contrary to fact—to be superb at minimizing the cost of the services he performs for his patients, the full extent of economies of scale from using ancillary personnel are attained in groups of small size—that is, the cost per patient visit falls as the group increases to three or four physicians, but not thereafter.

On methodological grounds, the most satisfactory studies of economies of scale in medical practice have been those of Ernst and Schwartz.[8] Unlike most researchers, they defined total practice cost to consist of: (1) tax deductible expenses (e.g., rent, salaries for nurses and clerks); (2) the cost of physician-owned assets (an estimate of the cost of renting assets, rather than an accounting estimate of depreciation of that equipment); and most important, (3) the cost of the physician's own time based on an estimate of the cost of hiring a physician for the practice. Thus, the authors were able to estimate the cost per patient visit for all of the resources provided by a medical practice, including physician inputs.

Using sophisticated multiple regression analysis, Ernst and Schwartz in their first study found that in most *single specialty* practices—particularly in the more common specialties, such as general practice, internal medicine, pediatrics, and general surgery— solo practice is the optimal (least-cost) practice mode.[9] Economies of scale were found to exist only in the hospital-based specialties, such as radiology and anesthesiology.

The most serious criticism of all studies of economies of scale, including even the Ernst and Schwartz study just cited, is that they do not provide sufficient control for differences in the nature and quality of care provided in practice modes of various sizes. As previously noted, the patient visit is not an appropriate measure of physician output if small practices perform only physician examinations and simple tests and refer the patient to laboratories, radiology centers, and hospitals for more complicated procedures, while group practices provide comprehensive health care in-house for their patients. Moreover, since the high paid medical specialists with their more costly procedures tend to serve in group practices, the cost per patient visit should be higher in those practices.

To deal with these problems, Ernst and Schwartz conducted a second study in which they attempted to measure economies of scale while exercising control over the composition of services, physician characteristics, organizational features of the practice, and the structure of local medical markets.[10] In this study, they examined only *multispecialty*, fee-for-service group practices that provided comprehensive care. Among the principal findings in this important study is the following:

> Total costs per visit, essentially the sum of direct non-physician costs and physician labor costs per visit, appear to be lower at the 35-to-55 physician group size. Hence, the evidence suggests that lowest average production costs are achieved by groups of these sizes.[11]

Noting that only ten groups in the thirty-five to fifty-five physicians size category and only four groups in the over-fifty-five physicians category were observed in their national sample, the authors drew the conservative conclusion that "the evidence is compatible with the . . . hypothesis of constant average costs up to the 55-physician size of practice."[12] The four groups that were larger than fifty-five physicians per group all had much higher costs per visit than other groups in the study. That may be because they are less efficient, or perhaps because they also serve as very high quality, expensive regional referral clinics in the tradition of such institutions as the Mayo Clinic, the Cleveland Clinic, the Palo Alto Clinic, Boston's Lahey Clinic, and the Ochsner Clinic in New Orleans. One cannot tell from the Ernst and Schwartz study whether the latter possibility is the case.

The third and final major conclusion that can be drawn about economies of scale is that actual practice-size distribution is consistent with the empirical findings that have just been summarized. Single specialty and general practice groups (defined as groups comprised of 75 percent or more physicians in one specialty) are mainly three to seven physicians in size. By contrast, though most multispecialty groups have fewer than sixteen physicians, most physicians who are practicing in multispecialty groups are in groups with sixteen or more physicians.[13]

Moreover, the percent of specialists in single specialty groups exceeds 20 percent only for anesthesiologists, orthopedic surgeons, pathologists, and radiologists. With the exception of orthopedic surgeons, these are the specialties that have been found to be subject to economies of scale in single specialty groups. For other specialties it is not unusual for at least 15 percent of physicians to be engaged in multispecialty group practice. However, with the exception of radiology, no specialty has as many as 40 percent of physicians practicing in groups with three or more physicians. The one-to-two physician practice is the dominant mode in virtually all specialties.[14]

The conclusions reached from this review of the literature about the modest gains that are potentially available from economies of scale seem contrary to reports that some of the large group practices, such as Kaiser, are more efficient than mainstream medical practice. One widely reported set of data included in the report of the National Advisory Commission on Health Manpower in 1967 shows that Kaiser has lower per capita utilization of services and hence lower annual costs per patient than does mainstream medicine. These comparisons are shown in Table 6-3.

Table 6-3. Comparative Statistics for Kaiser and California, 1965

| | | *Kaiser* | | |
		Northern California	*Southern California*	*California*
1.	Hospital beds/1,000	1.73	1.66	3.39
1a.	Age Adjusted	1.91		3.39
2.	Hospital days/1,000	532	520	891
2a.	Age Adjusted	612	—	891
3.	Average Daily Cost of Hospitalization	$56.06	—	$63.48
4.	Average Length of Stay	6.6	6.0	6.5
5.	Annual Hospital Cost per Person	$29.82		$56.06
5a.	Age Adjusted	$34.30		$56.06
6.	Physicians/1,000	.925	.906	1.26
7.	Physician Visits per Person	4.63	—	4.91
8.	Per Capita Cost of Physician Services	$44.32	—	{ $67. { $88.
9.	Other Related Expenses per Capita	$ 7.69	—	$ 8.76
10.	Total Per Capita Expenses	$81.83	$83.87	{ 131.82 { 152.82

Source: National Advisory Commission on Health Manpower, *Report of the Commission,* 2 vols., Washington, D.C., 1967, Vol. 2, p. 209.

It should be noted, however, that these data compare a *prepaid* group practice with *mainstream fee-for-service* practice modes. But economies of scale deal with the purely technical question of whether a particular medical service can be delivered at a lower cost in a large setting than in a small setting. Prepayment and fee-for-service, on the other hand, are financial arrangements for collecting revenues from patients. The advantages of Kaiser over mainstream practice are caused by the incentives under its prepaid financial system, not by economies of scale. Quoting the National Advisory Commission on Health Manpower:

> The study group [did not] find evidence of major innovations in the practice of medicine; Kaiser physicians use standard medical practices and procedures during their contacts with patients and there does not appear to be unusual substitution of auxiliary personnel for physicians. Neither do economies of scale associated with Kaiser's large group practices appear to be a major explanatory factor of the savings Kaiser achieves in providing medical care... if this is the case, what are the sources of economy? In the final analysis, it is the individual physician who has the most influence on the cost of medical care.... Kaiser has been able to achieve substantial savings because it has been able to get individual physicians to control the costs of providing medical care.[15]

In concluding this discussion of economies of scale, it should be stressed that this subject focuses exclusively on the important question of cost per patient. In principle, all other factors should be held constant while comparisons of cost per patient are made. In fact, practices of varying size differ considerably in terms of the care they provide and, perhaps, in the quality of that care. As Ernst and Schwartz have stated the issue:

> ...there may be benefits or costs to consumers from given scales of practice that are not directly related to the costs of or prices paid for physicians' services. These benefits or costs, measured in terms of accessibility, convenience, and patient satisfaction with the mode of delivery, may imply socially optimal scales of practice that do not minimize average production costs.[16]

The issues concerning economies of scale deserve to be debated in their own right. This review of our present knowledge of the issues, however, indicates that neither solo practice nor group practice is technically more efficient than the other.

Perhaps a case can be made that quality of care is more easily achieved (or less easily achieved) in large practice settings than in small. That is largely a medical question. From the evidence currently available, however, neither those who prefer small-scale practice nor those who advocate an expansion of practice size can legitimately use cost of care as an argument to support their particular preference.

Part IV

Incentives in
Medical Practice

Chapter Seven

Comparison of Practice Modes

Having decided on his specialty and perhaps on his geographic location while still in training, the physician's first
step in his transition into the world of practice is a crucial
decision that will profoundly affect his future earnings and professional life style. He must choose a practice mode, and, in making that
choice, he must weigh a number of factors related to the various
incentives inherent in each type of practice.

Doctors have five choices: (1) solo practice, (2) association, (3) fee-
for-service group practice, (4) prepaid group practice, and (5) salaried
positions.

SOLO PRACTICE

The solo practitioner owns and operates his own medical practice. He
is responsible for the health care of his patients. He shares this responsibility with other physicians only on a referral basis for specialty care or through informal agreements to take turns being on
call during nonoffice hours. Patients pay him on a fee-for-service
basis for the health care service he renders. In the case of general
practitioners and specialists in internal medicine and pediatrics, the
doctor provides continuing care as the "personal physician." Surgical
specialists provide short-term care for specific problems, but continuing care remains with the referring physicians.

The principal advantage to the physician in solo practice is independence. The solo practitioner has total discretion over patient
load, office hours, fees, and office management. Medical decisions

are his alone. Personality conflicts in his office practice are kept to a minimum, since the staff is small and subject to his control. His dealings with other physicians can be friendly and relaxed. He has complete freedom to determine to whom he will refer his patients and, hence, he can limit his referrals to physicians with whom he is friendly and whom he respects professionally. Finally, the solo practitioner has the satisfaction of knowing that his practice is something he has built and maintained on his own.

One necessary disadvantage that accompanies this independence is isolation. The solo practitioner is isolated in a number of ways. One of the most important is financial isolation. He alone incurs the cost of establishing and maintaining his practice. Because he works alone, another disadvantage of solo practice is that the doctor has less un-interrupted free time than physicians in other practice modes. In this regard, solo practitioners may trade calls with one another on week-ends, but usually they must handle their own calls during week nights. In rural areas where other physicians may not be available, they sometimes must be on call twenty-four hours a day, seven days a week. Thus, even though the solo practitioner does not spend more hours seeing patients than other doctors,[1] he typically spends more time on call than doctors in other practice modes.

Professional isolation is another important disadvantage of solo practice. The solo practitioner has no easy way to consult with other physicians. To be sure, he may refer his patients to another doctor; but he does not have access to informal consultation with immedi-ately available colleagues. He will also find it more difficult than other doctors to leave his patients to attend medical conferences, seminars, and other programs that doctors utilize to stay abreast of medical advances.

In addition to the disadvantages of isolation, solo practitioners tend to earn less money than doctors in all but the very large group practices.[2] One reason is that they are frequently in specialties where physicians earn less money—that is, general practice, pediatrics, and internal medicine. Another is that there are sometimes financial ad-vantages to group practice, as is shown later in the discussion of this practice mode.

ASSOCIATIONS

An association is an agreement of two or more doctors to share some expenses but otherwise to operate as fee-for-service solo practition-ers. For example, two internists may share the cost of rent, office furnishings, a receptionist, utilities, and janitorial services. But in every other way—setting of office hours, determination of fees, records keeping, billing and collection, and payroll—they might decide to operate completely separate practices. Hence, an association is a practice mode somewhere in between solo practice and group practice.

In an association, the doctor has some of the advantages of fee-for-service group practice: easily available consultation, coverage for calls, and even the ability to share in the cost of some expensive equipment that would not be economically feasible for the solo practitioner. At the same time, each doctor in an association has many of the advantages of the solo practitioner, such as independence and the knowledge that his income depends entirely on how hard he works and not on the productivity of other physicians. As contrasted with more formal group practice arrangements, their informal ties mean that associates will find it relatively easy to get along with one another.

FEE-FOR-SERVICE GROUP PRACTICE

Fee-for-service group practice occurs when two or more physicians organize formally to provide medical care through the joint use of personnel and equipment. All expenses are shared by the group members. Patients are billed by the group on a fee-for-service basis, and, unlike solo practices and associations, patients make their payments to the group, not to any specific physician in the group. The income of the group is then divided among the physicians according to some formula they have agreed upon. One formula calls for each doctor to take an equal share of the profits, perhaps after the group has set aside some money to be reinvested in the business. Other methods of dividing the profits include prorating them according to physician productivity—for example, the doctor's pay may be related to his contribution to the group's revenue. When a new physician joins a group, he usually works for a salary or for less than a full share of the profits until he begins to contribute a full share to the practice.

The advantages of fee-for-service group practice are of two types: professional and economic. The chief professional advantage is collegiality. Practicing medicine is lonely without other doctors, especially when the doctor is faced with difficult cases. Group practice provides an opportunity to consult easily with other physicians, and, as a result, the physician may be able to practice better medicine. Group practices often are able to purchase diagnostic and therapeutic equipment and services that would be uneconomical in a smaller medical setting. Moreover, if the group is large enough to hire a business manager, the physician will also be spared many of the details of running a medical practice. This freedom permits him to concentrate on the practice of medicine.

The most obvious advantage of fee-for-service group practice is that physicians in this mode tend to earn higher incomes than physicians in other practice modes. Several reasons account for the higher incomes of group practice physicians.

First, groups, especially the larger groups, tend to include specialists who can command high fees and thus increase the average earnings of all the physicians in the group.

Second, in some kinds of groups there are economies of scale—that is, the cost per patient visit falls as the number of doctors in the group increases. For example, a group of radiologists can share expensive x-ray, cobalt, and linear accelerator equipment, as well as technicians, while they see a large volume of patients. A single radiologist with the same equipment and personnel as a group would not be able to maintain as large a flow of patients. The total cost per patient, therefore, is smaller in the group setting.

Third, physicians in fee-for-service groups earn more money because the size of their combined practices makes it profitable for them to offer services usually available only on referral in solo practices. For example, a group may purchase x-ray equipment and laboratory facilities and do their own diagnostic work for their patients rather than send it to outside laboratories and x-ray facilities. The economic advantage to the doctor in such a group is that the group members earn the profit rather than radiologists, pathologists, commercial laboratories, and hospitals.

A fourth reason doctors earn higher income in fee-for-service groups goes to the heart of the economics of multispecialty group practice. To understand this point, consider a primary care physician and a specialist who obtains his patients on referral. Suppose the primary care physician is a general practitioner and the other doctor is a surgeon. The general practitioner is in a powerful position because the surgeon depends on general practitioners to refer business to him. The surgeon is also in a powerful position, however, because he is able to charge much higher fees for an hour of work than is the general practitioner. That is due in part to the fact that the demand for surgery is not much affected by the prices charged by surgeons. Probably more important, a special mystique surrounds surgery, which, in the public mind, justifies high surgical fees.

A profitable but unethical way for the general practitioner and the surgeon to do business together is as follows: The general practitioner refers a patient to the surgeon for a gall bladder operation. The surgeon performs the operation and charges a high fee, which the patient (with the help of his insurance company) gratefully pays. The surgeon gives part of the fee back to the general practitioner. This act is called *fee splitting*. It has been declared unethical by the American College of Surgeons, and it is illegal in a number of states. Nonetheless, it still occurs to some extent. A more subtle form of fee splitting is for the surgeon to invite the general practitioner to assist him in surgery and to participate in postoperative consultation. Sometimes the general practitioner's services are actually desired by the surgeon; other times the surgeon and the general practitioner are engaging in a form of make work or featherbedding.

Rather than making such arrangements unethically through fee splitting, however, the surgeon and the general practitioner can form a group and accomplish the same economic objectives ethically. Simply put, the group is a profitable replacement for fee splitting. The general practitioner and the other primary care physicians they invite to join their group will refer all their surgical patients to the group's surgeon. The surgeon will charge the usual high surgical fee, and the primary care physicians in the group will share with the surgeon in the fee paid by the patient.

Multispecialty group practice also solves another problem faced by primary physicians who are not in groups. Whenever they refer their patients to a physician outside their own practice, they not only lose the fee, they also run the risk of losing the patient. Of course, the specialist to whom the patient has been referred realizes that he must send the patient back if he is to continue to get referrals. But the patient himself may decide to drop the referring physician in favor of the specialist. In fee-for-service group practice, by contrast, the physician to whom the patient has been referred has little if any financial incentive to keep the patient, and even if the patient prefers to see the specialist more often after experiencing the referral, the referring physician is protected because all physicians in the group share in their collective profits.

In spite of the professional and economic advantages of fee-for-service groups, this practice mode also has its disadvantages. There are many problems stemming from personality clashes between doctors in the group. In addition to the problems faced in coordinating any organization, management of a group medical practice is complicated by the fact that the physicians in the group are roughly equal in status and autonomy.[3] Moreover, if one doctor in a group comes to believe that one of his colleagues is not particularly competent or that he is not working as hard as others in the group to contribute to the profits of the practice, then conflict is likely to be intense. Whether or not the doctors' spouses get along well with one another and with the members of the group can also have a strong impact on the success of the practice. Younger doctors in groups often resent the political influence of the senior doctors, and the senior doctors who founded the group are likely to resent the influence of newer doctors or to be jealous of the ease with which the younger doctors are able to begin to earn incomes the older doctors did not realize until late in their practice years. Finally, since very few doctors understand much about business, they are likely to have some troubles over money; even though fee-for-service group practice can be a profitable means of controlling referrals, physicians nonetheless may have serious problems over how to divide the profits they earn.

PREPAID GROUP PRACTICE

Although only a small percentage of doctors in this country practice in prepaid groups, many health care planners consider this practice mode to be the best hope for reform of the health care delivery system. Group practices with prepayment plans—Kaiser Permanente in the western states is one of the best known examples—contract with a group of people to provide medical care for a predetermined fee. Usually the fee is calculated on a per capita basis. For example, a trade union or a school district might contract with Kaiser for the health care of its members and their families. Kaiser would receive a fixed amount of income per year for each family, in return for which it would provide complete care with only nominal additional charges per patient visit.

An important advantage of this practice mode is that the doctor is typically able to work regular hours; once his shift is over, he need not be bothered with after-hours calls because someone else in the group is on duty. Under the prepaid group system, the doctor is usually freed of the responsibilities of management so that he can concentrate his entire attention on the practice of medicine. Moreover, he will often have a staff of allied health workers who free him to concentrate on those aspects of health care that require the attention of a physician. Finally, he has immediate access to colleagues for consultation, and usually the best diagnostic and therapeutic equipment and services are at his disposal.

The major disadvantage of prepaid group practice is financial. Doctors in prepaid groups tend to earn somewhat less than doctors in the fee-for-service practice modes, although the difference is not great except for the highest earners within the fee-for-service system.

Another disadvantage is that prepaid plans may offer a more impersonal style of health care delivery. Consequently, the doctor-patient relationship can be weaker in prepaid group practice than in fee-for-service practices, especially as compared with patients and primary care physicians in general practice, internal medicine, and pediatrics. Physicians who practice in prepaid groups may lose some status in the eyes of their patients and their fee-for-service medical colleagues. The former probably occurs because some people believe that the only doctors who would be willing to work in prepaid group practice are those who cannot succeed in the more lucrative fee-for-service mode. The latter may stem from the fact that many physicians resent the political and economic threat that prepaid practice represents to their professional and economic status; hence, they have a personal incentive to find fault with prepaid group practice and to criticize the physicians who practice in this mode.

SALARIED POSITIONS

Many young doctors accept salaried positions with group practices and hospitals upon completion of their training. They usually do so on a temporary basis to save the funds necessary to settle debts incurred during training and to finance the beginning of a private practice. Other physicians accept salaried positions with the government, typically to settle military obligations and occasionally to begin military careers. In 1974, the proportion of physicians employed by the federal government was 7.0 percent, approximately the same as it had been ten years earlier.[4]

Physicians in occupational health care generally work for large corporations and receive salaries and benefits typical of high-level management. The salaries for these positions vary as widely as do the earnings of private practitioners, but would generally be 10 to 25 percent lower than those of comparable specialists with similar backgrounds working in any of the other practice modes.

PRACTICE MODES IN THE UNITED STATES

Table 7-1 shows the status of group practice in the United States. In 1975 there were 8,483 group practices in the United States with 66,842 physicians. Group practice accounted for 23.5 percent of nonfederal physicians in 1975, compared with 17.6 percent in 1969.[5] This leaves 76.5 percent of nonfederal physicians who were practicing in one- or two-doctor offices in 1975, down from 82.4 percent in 1969.

Table 7-1.   Group Practices and Group Practice Physicians by Size and Type of Group, 1975

Type of Group	All Sizes	Size of Group					
		3-4	*5-7*	*8-15*	*16-25*	*26-49*	*50 & Over*
All Groups	8,483	4,437	2,284	1,148	326	187	101
Single Specialty	4,601	2,824	1,255	465	43	7	7
General Practice	906	661	196	41	6	2	0
Multispecialty	2,976	952	833	642	277	178	94
All Physicians	66,842	15,291	13,107	11,828	6,363	6,463	13,790
Single Specialty	23,572	9,831	7,087	4,554	807	206	1,087
General Practice	3,959	2,287	1,077	385	113	97	0
Multispecialty	39,311	3,173	4,943	6,889	5,443	6,160	12,703

Source: American Medical Association, J. R. Cantwell, ed., *Profile of Medical Practice, 1975-76* (Chicago: Center for Health Services Research and Development, American Medical Association, 1976), p. 11. Reprinted by permission of the American Medical Association.

Table 7-2.   Growth Rates of Number of Group Practices and Group Practice Physicians, 1969 to 1975

Type of Group	All Sizes	Size of Group					
		3-4	*5-7*	*8-15*	*16-25*	*26-49*	*50 & Over*
All Groups	33.15%	7.0%	73.69%	86.36%	111.69%	92.78%	102.00%
Single Specialty	45.19	18.66	96.09	232.14	514.29	250.00	N/A
General Practice	15.56	-7.94	221.31	720.00	N/A		N/A
Multispecialty	23.08	-8.55	35.67	36.31	88.44	87.37	88.00
All Physicians	66.72	10.32	77.00	86.97	108.35	96.62	123.83
Single Specialty	80.59	23.80	97.93	239.60	530.47	207.46	N/A
General Practice	47.12	-1.63	236.56	736.96	N/A	N/A	N/A
Multispecialty	61.45	-11.71	40.87	39.48	86.02	91.30	106.18

Source: American Medical Association, J. R. Cantwell, ed., *Profile of Medical Practice, 1975-76* (Chicago: Center for Health Services Research and Development, American Medical Association, 1976), p. 12. Reprinted by permission of the American Medical Association.

Table 7-2 shows the growth rates of group practices of various sizes. Single specialty groups are growing fastest in the eight or more physician group sizes, general practice groups are growing rapidly in the eight to fifteen physician category, and the multispecialty groups are growing most rapidly in the sixteen or more physicians group practices. (In this table, groups with 75 percent or more of their physicians in the same specialty are classified as single-specialty groups or as general practice groups.)

There were 385 prepaid group practices in the United States in 1969 and 713 in 1975, an increase of 80 percent. The greatest number of these groups receive less than 5 percent of their income from prepaid practice; the remainder comes from fee-for-service practice. Only 21 percent receive at least half of their revenues from prepaid practice.[6]

Clearly, then, the one- or two-man office remains the choice of the majority of active physicians. But the advantages of group practice organization—collegiality and after-hours coverage, combined with financial considerations—are likely to continue to erode the prominent position of solo practice in American medicine.

Chapter Eight

Physician Earnings and Medical Fees

No occupational category in the United States earns more than physicians. Table 8-1 shows the most recent data available on gross income, expenses, and net income of American physicians.

Gross income in 1974 averaged more than $85,000 per year for all physicians and surpassed $100,000 for some surgical specialties. It

Table 8-1. Average Income of U.S. Physicians by Specialty, 1974

	*Gross**	*Expenses*	*Net*
All Physicians	$ 86,575	$35,351	$51,224
General Practice	80,738	36,930	43,808
Internal Medicine	88,094	36,979	51,115
Surgeon	101,597	41,566	60,031
Obstetrics-gynecology	100,010	41,772	58,238
Pediatrics	78,790	35,361	43,429
Psychiatry	55,224	15,227	39,997
Anesthesiology	67,092	16,312	50,780

*Figures in this column were computed by the authors.

Source: American Medical Association, J. R. Cantwell, ed., *Profile of Medical Practice, 1975-76* (Chicago: Center for Health Services Research and Development, American Medical Association, 1976), pp. 154 and 164. Reprinted by permission of the American Medical Association.

should be noted, however, that the physician, regardless of his specialty, incurs large costs in the operation of his business. The average net income—income after expenses—of American physicians was

83

about $51,000 in 1974. Only surgeons averaged net income as large as $60,000.

Figure 8-1 shows that physicians vary widely in their pretax incomes, with some earning considerably more than the national average of $51,000, and others much less. In 1974 about 22 percent of U.S. physicians had a net income of $30,000 per year or less. On the high-income end of the earnings spectrum, another 28 percent earned more than $60,000 per year, and 18 percent earned in excess of $70,000. The middle range of physicians (50 percent), however, earned between $30,000 and $60,000 per year.

FIGURE 8-1. Percentage Distribution of U.S. Physicians by Net Income, Estimated for 1974.

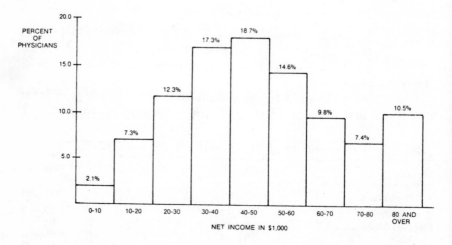

Source: American Medical Association, J. R. Cantwell, ed., *Profile of Medical Practice, 1975-76* (Chicago: Center for Health Services Research and Development, American Medical Association, 1976), p. 162. Reprinted by permission of the American Medical Association.

An estimate of the distribution of gross incomes can be inferred from Figure 8-1 by multiplying the net income figures by 1.7. For the "70,000 and over" categories in Figure 8-1, we can estimate that almost 18 percent of physicians have gross earnings of more than $120,000 per year ($71,000 x 1.7 = $120,000).

Although physician incomes are quite high compared with those of the population as a whole, most physicians nevertheless do not earn enough to become wealthy. Many businessmen have incomes vastly larger than those of physicians.

One should note that the net earnings in Table 8-1 and Figure 8-1 include few fringe benefits. Most doctors must provide for their own accident, health and life insurance, as well as for their retirement. Reported net earnings are also pretax, and physicians have few effective ways of obtaining tax exclusions and deductions to reduce their income taxes. They may claim all the usual deductions, such as interest on their homes, and they are permitted to deduct business-related travel expenses, which often include a large percentage of the cost of an expensive car and expenditures for attending medical meetings. Beyond these possibilities, the physician has little to claim except business expenses for his often unsuccessful outside investments.

Finally, few occupations require a person to train so long before beginning to earn at peak levels as medicine does. Not many physicians complete their training before the age of thirty, and, as Table 8-2 shows, doctors in many specialties do not reach their peak earning years until after age forty.

Table 8-2. Average Net Income by Age of Physician and Specialty, Estimated 1974

	Specialty					
Age	*General Practice*	*Internal Medicine*	*Surgery*	*Obstetrics-Gynecology*	*Pediatrics*	*Psychiatry*
Total	$43,772	$51,125	$60,155	$58,270	$43,422	$39,957
35 and under	53,978	40,929	46,125	55,857	31,148	42,636
36-40	49,344	53,925	63,541	61,019	48,868	37,623
41-45	50,921	61,648	67,429	65,636	51,667	44,667
46-50	54,065	62,417	69,274	68,471	43,574	42,574
51-60	44,487	50,447	65,097	57,560	43,522	40,530
61 and over	30,706	41,098	43,827	36,778	33,586	30,327

Source: American Medical Association, J. R. Cantwell, ed., *Profile of Medical Practice, 1975-76* (Chicago: Center for Health Services Research and Development, American Medical Association, 1976), p. 171. Reprinted by permission of the American Medical Association.

Over the period 1969-1974 physician net incomes failed to grow as fast as their practice expenses, despite substantial increases in physician fees. Average expenses increased from $21,000 per year in 1969 to $35,000 in 1974, a compound growth rate of 10.7 percent. Physicians responded by raising their fees. The average fee for an initial office visit increased from $12.80 in 1969 to $19.55 in 1974, a compound growth rate of 8.8 percent. Consequently, net income from medical practice grew at only 5.2 percent in rising from $40,000 in 1969 to $51,000 in 1974. Federal price controls that were imposed on the health care industry from August 1971 through April 1974 appear to be the major cause of these trends. Sufficient data are not yet available to determine what has happened to physician incomes since 1974. Physician fees have been rising sharply since controls were removed. Some of this increase may reflect the attempt of physicians to make up for the effects of controls. On the other hand, increases in costs, especially the well-publicized increases in malpractice insurance rates, work to undermine the physician's economic position.

Rather than focusing on annual income, one can more effectively evaluate physician earnings by answering the following question: What rate of return does a person earn by investing his money in a medical education? Studies by economists indicate that, after allowing for expenses and earnings foregone while training, physicians realize an average return of 12 percent on their investment in a medical education.[1] Some studies indicate that specialty training may actually yield a negative rate of return.[2] The average rate of return on business investment in the United States is about 12 percent. Thus physicians appear to realize no greater return on their investment in medical training than do investors in other types of business. They do, however, invest more time and money in their training than most people, and this high investment eventually provides them with earnings greater than those of individuals in many other occupations.

PRICING OF MEDICAL SERVICES

In the past, before third-party payments through insurance companies and the government became commonplace, the individual physician exercised considerable discretion and independence in fee setting. Sometimes he charged different prices to different patients, depending on their ability to pay.[3] In determining what he would charge for each service, he also tended to bill patients according to their willingness to pay. Since willingness to pay is strongly correlated with the nature of a patient's medical problem, physicians in some specialties were able to charge more for an hour of their time than were others.

The rise of third-party private insurance and the enactment of government programs to pay the bills of the elderly and the poor have led to important changes in the way physicians price their services. For one thing, most physicians no longer set different fees for different patients as they once did. Today, for any given procedure, the physician typically charges the same fee to all patients. This charge is called his usual, customary, and reasonable (UCR) fee. The insurance carriers and the government, however, are not alway willing to compensate physicians for their UCR fees because to do so would encourage physicians to raise their fees to increase their incomes. Instead, insurance programs often specify some maximum allowable fee that they will pay for the various procedures that the physician performs for his insured patients.

To simplify physician billing of insurance companies, classification systems have been established to permit easy identification of the many procedures performed by physicians. On his billing, rather than write a full description of the care he provided a particular patient, a physician can identify that procedure by using a code number. State medical societies have helped to simplify third-party billing by developing classification codes that can be used by all physicians in the state.

A logical next step has been for physicians to use these classification codes to reach some agreement about the relative value of the various procedures they perform. The California Medical Association was the first to develop such a relative value scale (RVS). To illustrate its use, a "brief evaluation" is assigned a unit value of 20, a "comprehensive evaluation" a unit value of 70, and a "cardiac catheterization" a unit value of 350.[4] California physicians, if they wish, may use the relative value scale to determine their fees simply by selecting a dollar multiplier. Physicians who select a multiplier of $1.00 would, therefore, charge $20 for a brief evaluation, $70 for a comprehensive evaluation, and $350 for a cardiac catheterization.

Other state medical societies and the societies of some medical specialties, following the lead of the California Medical Association, have also developed relative value scales. Although no one knows what proportion of physicians determine their fees by applying a dollar multiplier to some relative value scale, all indications are that the practice is very widespread.

The unit values in a relative value scale can be established in more than one way. One method would be to base unit values on the amount of physician time a procedure takes—that is, if one procedure takes fifteen minutes and another a half-hour, the latter could be assigned twice as many points. The fee schedule used until recently by Workers' Compensation in California is one example of

Table 8–3.   California Relative Value Studies (RVS) Code—Physician Payment Schedules, 1976

RVS Code	Physician Service	Usual, Customary and Reasonable (UCR)	Medical Care Foundation	Workers' Compensation	Medicare	Medicaid (Medi-Cal)
90000	Brief Evaluation	$ 20–30	$ 22.00	$ 20.65	$ 20.00	$ 12.30
90020	Comprehensive Evaluation	65–80	77.00	61.25	59.00	36.90
90040	Brief Follow-up	15–20	16.00	12.25	14.00	6.15
90060	Intermediate Follow-up	20–30	22.00	22.75	15.00	12.30
90250	Hospital Visit	18–30	22.00	18.20	17.70	12.30
90600	Limited Consultation	30–40	33.00	34.65	35.00	18.45
90620	Comprehensive Consultation	70–90	77.00	77.00	70.00	43.05
49503	Bilateral Hernia Repair	550–650	522.50	520.00	400.00	307.50
58150	Total Hysterectomy	800–1000	880.00	—	700.00	369.00
44950	Appendectomy	500–600	522.50	—	400.00	246.00
71020	Chest X-Ray	25–30	25.80	26.60	22.00	18.45
70260	Skull X-Ray Series	50–60	51.60	49.70	41.00	30.75
93000	Electrocardiogram	25–35	30.00	28.00	21.00	18.45

such a system.[5] But this approach does not take into account costs that are not directly related to physician time. For example, some procedures require specialized equipment while others require special materials or the deployment of physician aides. The degree of risk, and hence the likelihood that the physician will be sued for malpractice, also varies according to the kind of procedure being performed. Developing a relative value scale to take all such costs into account can be difficult and controversial.

Consequently, some relative value scales are based on typical physician fees rather than on some estimate of physician time or costs. The unit values of the California Medical Association RVS, for example, are computed by calculating median physician fees. Thus, if surgeons typically charge twice as much for a nasal bone graft as for a bilateral mastectomy, the bone graft is given a unit value twice that of the mastectomy.

Physicians in some specialties earn more than those in other specialties because patients are willing to pay more for some services than for others. Health insurance also covers a larger proportion of the fees of some specialists than others. Thus, surgeons typically can charge more per hour than can pediatricians. Perhaps to downplay such differences in fees among the various specialties, the California Medical Association in its relative value scale reports unit values in a way that makes it impossible for the physician to compare the relative value of procedures in medicine, anesthesia, surgery, radiology, and pathology. Unit values are comparable within each classification, but not across classifications.

Differences in the extent to which health insurance carriers and government programs reimburse physicians create important incentives. Table 8-3 shows thirteen medical services commonly provided by physicians. For purposes of illustration, the five-digit identification code of the California Medical Association's Relative Value Studies code is shown for each procedure. The charges shown in this table are typical of those found in the San Francisco Bay Area in 1976. The first column shows a range of fees considered to be "usual, customary, and reasonable" by physicians in fee-for-service practice. These amounts are billed to patients who pay cash for medical care or who have insurance through Blue Shield or other independent health insurance companies. The physician bills the patient at his UCR rate, and the insurance company reimburses all or a part of the bill. The patient may be held responsible for that part of the bill not covered by insurance. Physicians have a strong incentive to see patients who can be billed at their UCR rates. In fact, because of the certainty of being paid by Blue Shield and other health insurance companies, the insured patient is frequently preferred to the patient who promises to pay the full UCR fee out of his own pocket but who might also become a collection problem for the physician.

The second column shows the fees charged by physician members of a medical care foundation. A medical care foundation is a decentralized group practice run by members of a county medical society. In this example, the foundation negotiates fees with groups of patients, for example, the members of a trade union. Members of the trade union receive their care from office-based physicians who belong to the foundation, and the physicians are paid at the negotiated rates. Physicians like to have patients whose care is provided under medical care foundation contracts. The negotiated fees they receive usually are comfortably within the range of UCR fees, and they have no problems in collecting them.

The third column shows rates from the *Official Minimum Medical Fee Schedule* used to reimburse California physicians for patients insured by Workers' Compensation. Industrial injuries preinsured by the Workers' Compensation Insurance Program are paid on a fee-for-service basis, but reimbursement rates are set individually by each state. Typically, these rates are on the low side of the range of fee schedules. (The rates shown here reflect a recent increase to bring them closer to UCR fees, below which they had been allowed to drop by a substantial amount.) As might be expected, the lower rate of payment discourages busy physicians from welcoming industrial illnesses and injuries into their private offices.

Physician services provided under the Medicare program for eligible patients over the age of 65 are reimbursed in accordance with an "economic index factor." The economic index is calculated annually and reflects the changes that have been taking place in physicians' practice expenses and in physician earning levels since 1971. However, cumbersome delays in adjusting Medicare fees upward, while holding down the cost of this program to the taxpayer, also make the Medicare patient less attractive to the physician than the patient who pays the full UCR fee. Physicians who accept "assignment" of Medicare patients are not permitted to bill these patients for the difference between the UCR fee and the amount allowed by Medicare. Consequently, some doctors do not treat Medicare patients unless they are also covered by supplemental insurance, in which case the physician may bill the patient for the difference between what Medicare allows and the UCR fee. The incentive to turn away Medicare patients increases as the gap between what the physician bills and what Medicare allows is permitted to grow.

The last column shows payments made in California under the Medicaid program. Medicaid is designed to provide health care benefits to the poor. This program is administered by the states, and benefits vary considerably from one state to another. In general, however, the rates of reimbursement are so far below the physicians' UCR fees that physicians who can keep their practices occupied by seeing other categories of patients have a strong financial incentive to do so. Hence, Medicaid patients are often relegated to public hospitals or to medical practices that see them on a high-volume basis. The result is that a second and inferior system of health care is created for the poor. In some places Medicaid "mills" have been created in which unscrupulous doctors give inadequate care and defraud the government.

Relative value scales provide a convenient avenue for local physicians to engage in price fixing. Furthermore, "ethics" of the medical community encourage physicians to "keep their prices in line" with those of their fellow physicians. Government programs and insurance company reimbursement practices also foster this attitude. The government's antitrust lawyers have recognized the potential of relative value schedules to be used in price fixing. In November 1975, the Justice Department filed an antitrust suit against the American Society of Anesthesiologists for violation of the Sherman Antitrust Act. The suit attacks relative value schedules by claiming that their use by anesthesiologists amounts to a conspiracy to "raise, fix, stabilize, and maintain fees. . . ." The consequence of the alleged conspiracy, says the government, is that fees have been maintained at "artificial and noncompetitive levels" and that such prices deny to patients purchasing anesthesia services "the right to obtain such services at competitively determined fees." In July of 1976 the American Academy of Orthopaedic Surgeons and the American College of Obstetricians and Gynecologists signed consent decrees agreeing to abandon their relative value scales. The legality of relative value scales will undoubtedly be determined by the courts.[6]

Physician peer pressure, relative value scales, and the payment practices of insurance companies and the government all encourage physicians to gravitate toward common fees. The physician who charges either less or more than the "legitimate" fee being charged by the majority of doctors in his area is made to feel unethical.

One additional consequence under such a system, unfortunately, is that there is no way in which superior quality can be rewarded and inferior quality penalized. With common prices, physician earnings are determined by one factor only, that factor being patient volume. It necessarily follows that a physician of poor quality with a large practice made up of patients with whom he spends limited amounts of time can easily outstrip the earnings of the finest of physicians practicing the very highest quality of medicine.

Chapter Nine

The Effect of Incentives
on Health Care

Decisions by patients to seek medical care and decisions by physicians concerning the quality and quantity of that care appear to be fairly straightforward: The patient with a medical complaint seeks the help of a physician, and the physician provides health care according to generally accepted medical standards. Closer examination, however, makes evident that these decisions are not straightforward at all; rather, they are influenced in important ways by the financial incentives offered both patients and physicians. To understand the ultimate effect of financial incentives in medicine on the health care system and health care costs, one must first determine what those incentives are, how they vary from one practice mode to another, the effect of the fee-for-service payment mechanism on the incentives of both patients and physicians, and, finally, the differences between incentives in the fee-for-service mode and those in prepaid group practice.

PATIENT INCENTIVES

Analyzing a person's incentives requires first an understanding of what that person is trying to accomplish—that is, knowledge about his objectives. Although much has been written on this subject by economists and psychologists, scholars still disagree about it. For present purposes, however, one can assume that a person strives chiefly to promote the well-being of himself and the members of his family. In the economic sphere, to attain a state of well-being people consume goods and services. Since disposable income is always too small to permit the individual person to purchase everything that he wants, each must choose how he will spend his income from the wide range of alternative goods and services that are available. The outcome of such decisions depends heavily on the prices of the goods and services and on the person's income. Purchase decisions related to medical care are no exception.

Good health is important because it contributes to an individual's well-being in many ways. The influence of health on economic well-being is especially important. The family breadwinner's good health is crucial to the entire family since the family income may be cut off if he or she becomes ill. Health problems for anyone in the family, moreover, can lead to medical bills that impose severe financial strains on the family; to pay medical bills, income must be diverted from other purchases and sometimes savings and other assets must be depleted.

Fee-for-Service Health Care

In the United States, the most common payment mechanism for health care is fee-for-service. Virtually all doctors in solo practice, in associations, and in group practices use this payment system exclusively. Under this system, the patient seeks out a doctor, receives medical care, and then is billed by the doctor or his group for that care.

When using the fee-for-service health care system, people protect themselves and their families against the financial consequences of poor health by purchasing health insurance. Such insurance protects the incomes of working members of the household as well as the family's financial assets. By paying medical bills, health insurance helps the family maintain its standard of living; it is also an effective protection against catastrophic illness and the financial obligations that such an illness can create.

Because of tax subsidies available to purchasers of health insurance, many families find purchasing medical care through health insurance cheaper than paying for it directly as the care is received. Under the personal income tax, one-half of the cost of premiums for health insurance up to $150 plus all health care expenses (including remaining premiums) in excess of 3 percent of income may be deducted on each tax return. In addition, employers' contributions to health insurance plans of their employees are not taxable as income. In 1974 the federal government lost an estimated $5.6 billion in tax revenues because of these subsidies. This is an amount comparable to the federal expenditures on Medicaid, and it represents 17 percent of the nation's payments for health insurance premiums.[1]

About 11 cents out of every group health insurance dollar goes to pay for the operation of health insurance plans. Taken by itself this would mean that medical care provided through health insurance costs more than when it is directly purchased. But the average tax subsidy is almost 17 percent of premiums. Thus, on average the cost of health care is 6 percent less if a family is insured. This advantage tends to increase with income, averaging more than 12 percent for families with incomes of $20,000-$50,000 and almost 27 percent for families with incomes of $50,000-$100,000.[2]

Almost two-thirds of health insurance is purchased indirectly by employers and unions as part of group benefit packages.[3] Virtually all group insurance (96 percent) is provided through employment-related groups.[4] Since the programs usually selected by employers or unions are designed to meet the needs of workers who have seniority and responsibilities, these programs probably provide more health insurance than younger workers with fewer family obligations would need or be willing to purchase. Thus, such group health insurance probably overinsures one segment of the American people.[5]

The person who has health insurance has a financial incentive to obtain health care services more often than the individual who has no insurance. This situation exists because, for the insured person, out-of-pocket expenses for medical care at the time it is provided are typically small compared with the total cost of the care received. To guard against excessive utilization of health care services, health insurance companies typically control costs by specifying that their policies will cover only certain types of care or only a fraction of the cost of some categories of care. For example, health insurance companies commonly pay for hospital care but not for visits to doctors' offices or for hospital care received as an outpatient.

Unfortunately, this technique for reducing the incentive of patients to overutilize the health care system creates additional incentives for patients to distort their use of health care. Thus, they may pressure their physicians to hospitalize them rather than treat them as outpatients, so that the insurance company will pay the bill. All too often, the physician agrees because his own incentives are more compatible with those of the patient than those of the insurance company. The cost of the "hotel" service given to people in hospital beds—people who could just as well be at home were it not for the incentives created by insurance—are passed on to other health care consumers in the form of higher health insurance premiums and higher hospital bills.

Health insurance providers also try to control the excessive utilization of health care services by requiring that patients pay part of their medical bills. Unfortunately, the disincentive effect created by this approach has its greatest impact on the poor. Too often, this requirement keeps the poor from seeking health care until they are seriously ill when the cost of treating them can be greater than if they had sought care earlier.[6]

Martin S. Feldstein, an economist at Harvard University, has considered a related problem. The effect of prepaying health care through private and government insurance may be to give an incentive to hospitals to provide a more expensive product to health care consumers than they actually wish to purchase. Because the consumer's out-of-pocket cost at the time of illness is small, he may be willing to buy more expensive care than if he were not insured. This incentive can be as important for affluent families with substantial assets as for low-income families with few savings. The result is that the production of high-cost hospital care is a self-reinforcing process. As Feldstein puts it, "people spend more on health because they are insured and buy more insurance because of the high cost of health care."[7]

Prepaid Health Care

In most respects, the incentives of members of prepaid health care plans are no different from those of their counterparts who utilize the fee-for-service practice mode. To some extent, however, members of prepaid practices have a stronger incentive to use health services than do patients of physicians in fee-for-service practices. After all, at the time that he considers seeking medical care, the member of a prepaid plan has virtually no direct out-of-pocket costs, whereas the fee-for-service patient must pay for that part of his medical bill not covered by his insurance.

Given that members of prepaid plans pay nothing, or virtually nothing, at the time of treatment, they could be expected to over-utilize prepaid plans for minor complaints. For most, however, the problem is controlled somewhat by other costs. People who are employed may lose wages when they leave work to obtain medical care; money for babysitters, the cost of travel, and the value of time spent in waiting rooms are also costs that members of prepaid plans must pay to obtain health care. Finally, physicians in well-conceived prepaid health plans have no financial incentives to encourage patients with psychosomatic complaints to seek medical attention or to visit doctors because they are lonely. Under the fee-for-service system, however, physicians have a financial interest in continuing to see such patients.

People have a somewhat greater incentive to seek preventive care under prepaid modes than they do under the fee-for-service system of health care because, under prepaid plans, money is not a barrier once the capitation is paid. The importance of this incentive, however, has probably been exaggerated. First, patients in the fee-for-service health care system can have their laboratory work and x-rays for periodic examinations paid for by their insurance companies, although to do so requires that the physician engage in some deception in completing the insurance forms. Second, many physicians, both in fee-for-service and in prepaid plans, doubt the efficacy of many types of periodic examinations (e.g., the annual physical examination). Consequently, physicians in prepaid plans are not likely to reinforce the wishes of their subscribers to have such medical services performed for them. Whatever the incentive, a generally conceded fact is that prepaid plans actually practice very little more, if any more, preventive medicine than do fee-for-service physicians.

PHYSICIAN INCENTIVES

Like the patient, the physician is a member of a household. Therefore, he also can be presumed to seek the well-being of himself and his family. Unlike his patients, however, many of the physician's desires are satisfied by the practice of medicine, and one of his strong drives is to ensure the well-being of his patients. Part of the fee-for-service physician's concern for his patients, to be sure, may be motivated by narrow self-interest—that is, if the doctor does not take proper care of his patients, they will seek care elsewhere and, if that happens, the doctor and his family will experience a decrease in their standard of living.

Except for the risk of hospitalization and long-term disability, the fee-for-service physician does not share with other people some of the financial risks of being unable to pay for health care because, as a professional courtesy, doctors treat other physicians and their families at no cost. Two strong financial incentives encourage this practice. The first is that caring for the family of other doctors strengthens the personal bonds among the doctors and, perhaps, among their families. This has the effect of strengthening the patient referral relationships among physicians. The second is that doctors realize income tax advantages from the practice. Suppose, in a given year, "Dr. Warner's" family receives $1,000 worth of care from other physicians, and he also gives $1,000 worth of care to the families of his colleagues. If the doctors were to pay one another for health care, "Dr. Warner" would be required to pay the income tax owed on his $1,000 worth of income, undoubtedly a larger amount than the taxes he would save by paying $1,000 to other doctors and deducting the expense on his tax return.

THE PHYSICIAN'S ROLE IN HEALTH CARE

In this century, the health care delivery system has evolved from the single physician providing total health care for a group of patients to a complicated system entailing high technology; hospitals, clinics, and laboratories; allied health personnel; and specialized physicians. As John H. Knowles of the Rockefeller Foundation has observed:

> The inexorable expansion of science and technology has resulted in necessary discontinuity of care, subdivision of labor, and increasing costs. What used to be a one patient–one doctor relationship is now one patient to one doctor to another doctor to fifteen to twenty people standing behind each doctor in the hospital and in other institutions related to health.[8]

Today, the physician practicing in fee-for-service medicine is not only a direct provider of services, but also a central figure in determining many other health care costs. He alone decides his patient's treatment, its duration, whether or not hospitalization is necessary, the drugs to be used, and which other types of physicians and medical personnel should share in the management of the problem. As a result, the physician's impact on total health care costs is profound. Thus, although only 18 percent of the medical dollar is spent on physician services as compared with 39 percent for hospital care and 9 percent for drugs,[9] the decisions of individual physicians determine most of the nation's health care bill.

Under the fee-for-service health care system, the physician serves as a purchasing agent for his patients. When the patient visits his physician with a problem, he is asking to be told what medical care he should purchase. The physician may prescribe diagnostic work, such as physical examinations, laboratory tests, x-rays, and consultation with other physicians, as well as therapeutic care ranging from diets and exercise programs to prescription drugs, physical therapy, surgery, radiation, and chemotherapy. The products and services that the physician prescribes for the patient will often include many that are supplied by other enterprises—for example, pharmacies, hospitals, medical laboratories, and physicians in various specialties.

At the American Medical Association 1974 Leadership Conference, health economist Barbara H. Kehrer, discussing the physician as a purchasing agent, stated:

Physicians make decisions all the time which affect the cost of medical care to the patient and the utilization of scarce medical resources but for which physicians themselves bear no financial responsibility. The following types of decisions which physicians make are reflected in their patients' medical bills and affect the way society's scarce resources are allocated in the provision of care:

the decision to *hospitalize* rather than to treat the patient on an out-patient basis, and the length of the period of hospitalization;

decisions regarding the *techniques* chosen for diagnosis including the ordering of tests, and the number and types of tests selected;

the decision to utilize one instead of several alternative means of *treating* a given condition or illness;

decisions regarding the prescription of *drugs:* which of several alternative drugs is prescribed, the prescribed dosage, and the quantity of the drugs ordered. . . .

It is true, of course, that there are many instances in which cost considerations would not properly enter into a physician's decisions. Our society has not reached a point at which it is considered proper to make cost-benefit decisions in determining whether or not an individual patient should receive an expensive life-saving set of treatments; nor would most people wish it to be so. But the physician can act more responsibly as his patient's purchasing agent without attempting to resolve such problems. The purchasing agent issue focuses attention on areas of *discretionary decision-making.* The physician probably has a reasonable amount of discretion in many instances with regard to alternative choices, where there is significant variation in the cost implications of each alternative but little variation in the quality of medical care rendered. Those who have tried to call attention to the purchasing agent role of the physician are saying that, in such instances, it is to the benefit of both the patient and society as a whole if the physician takes cost as well as medical implications of his decisions into account in treating his patients.[10]

A strong case can be made that physicians, acting as purchasing agents, frequently make inappropriate decisions for their patients, and many of these decisions result in the overtreatment of patients. This situation stems from the four main causes discussed in the following sections.

The Physician's Lack of Business Training

Physicians lack the background for making the financial decisions that must be made in the treatment of patients. They are not economists or financial planners or businessmen. They have no training in business and management. Yet, by the tens of thousands, they are making decisions each day that determine the cost of health care to the nation—a cost that now amounts to more than $120 billion per year. Despite this authority, physicians are most often unaware of the full economic impact of their decisions. The problem is further compounded by the increasing complexity of medicine today.

The Technologic Imperative

One of the basic traditions of medicine is that health care must be of the highest quality possible. As the Stanford economist Victor Fuchs has observed, this tradition "... emphasizes giving the best care technically possible"; it is a tradition in which "... the only legitimate and explicitly recognized constraint is the state of the art."[11] With today's advanced medical technology, the possibilities for abusing this tradition appear almost endless. Moreover, the tradition unfortunately ignores the principle that health care resources should not be committed unless the benefits to be gained from using these resources exceed the value that society would realize if they were used in some other way.

Defensive Medicine

Medical malpractice suits and the size of the monetary awards related to them have grown dramatically over the past few years. In California, for example, the number of malpractice claims filed increased from 13.5 per 100 physicians in 1965 to 18 per 100 physicians in 1975.[12] The average malpractice settlement is approximately $8,500, and jury verdicts now average more than $350,000. California has had a $4.5 million award, and awards of $1 million occur in that state about once a month.[13]

In most parts of the country, malpractice insurance premiums have gone up sharply. In some places, premiums increased by 500 percent in the years 1975 and 1976. In 1976, physicians paid premiums for insurance ranging from about $400 to more than $40,000, depending on geographic location and physician specialty. Coverage for surgical specialists is the most costly.

To protect themselves against the possibility of malpractice suits, some physicians are refusing to treat high-risk patients. Physicians also have a strong incentive to order more services—especially consultations with specialists, laboratory tests, and x-rays—than they believe their patients actually need. Former Secretary of Health, Education, and Welfare, Casper W. Weinberger, has stated that defensive medicine resulted in society's paying between $3 billion and $7 billion additional health care costs in 1975.[14] In 1976, the cost is probably substantially higher. Some experts think it may be as high as $15 billion.

Incentives toward Overtreatment in the Fee-for-Service Mode

The fee-for-service physician can never forget, no matter how ethical he is, that he earns a fee if he performs a service and he earns nothing if he does not. It is in marginal or borderline decisions where the physician is most likely to treat rather than not to treat his patient.

The fee-for-service incentive system also rewards those doctors who create a demand for their own services. Patients sometimes suspect their doctors of having provided extra health care upon learning that they were covered by health insurance. An emerging body of research supports the common public suspicion that at least some doctors, some of the time, engage in the creation of demand.[15]

By contrast, in prepaid plans, members pay the medical group a fixed amount per month, in return for which the health care plan is "at risk" to provide for all the health care needs of its subscribers. Because the profit of the plan is the difference between the prepaid fees and any expenses the plan incurs while treating members, the plan has an incentive to keep costs to a minimum.

Doctors under some prepaid plans receive a guaranteed salary. Therefore, the doctor's income does not depend on his selling his own services; he can consider good patient care without simultaneously being interested in increasing his income. An accompanying disadvantage, however, is that the physician in such prepaid plans may not have as strong an incentive to work hard seeing large numbers of patients or to make certain that his patients are happy about the care they are receiving.

Salaried physicians in prepaid plans are usually given an incentive to control costs and avoid overtreatment. To accomplish that, the management of such plans may provide bonuses to their salaried physicians, with the bonuses based on the profits of the plan or on some indicator of cost, such as the rate of hospitalization. Hence, the size of the doctor's bonuses depends on his ability to contain costs to the organization.

In most prepaid plans, rather than working for a salary, physicians operate "at risk"—that is, they are the ones who receive the capitation payment in return for providing care for subscribers, and the difference between revenue and expense is theirs. The incentive in these plans for physicians to avoid overtreatment is compelling.

AREAS OF PROLIFERATING COST IN
FEE-FOR-SERVICE PRACTICE

The incentives in fee-for-service practice have resulted in proliferating costs to the health care consumer. The primary problem areas, in this regard, are drug prescriptions, hospitalization, unnecessary laboratory tests and x-rays, and unneeded surgical procedures.

Drug Prescription

The physician frequently adds to the cost of health care for his patients by his method of prescribing medications. More than $10 billion per year is spent on the purchase of prescription drugs. Approximately 90 percent of physician prescriptions call for brand name products and only 10 percent specify generic products. Yet, generic drugs are less costly and are often reliable substitutes for their brand name counterparts. As noted by Milton Silverman and Philip Lee in *Pills, Profits, and Politics*, about 75 percent of the most frequently prescribed drugs on the market are under patent and can be obtained only from brand-name manufacturers.[16] Consequently, even if a physician prescribes a patented drug generically, his patient will receive the brand-name drug. Nonetheless, physicians have many opportunities to reduce the cost of drugs to the patient by prescribing generically those drugs that no longer have patent protection.

Why then do physicians so frequently neglect cost considerations when prescribing drugs? First, their income is not increased according to whether they prescribe low-cost generic drugs or the more expensive brand-name drugs. In fact, the physician who is dedicated to saving money for his patients will soon find that the time he spends poring over drug lists searching for the lowest cost items could be spent more profitably seeing patients.

Advertising also appears to be an important factor in the doctor's approach to drug prescription. The Food and Drug Administration has estimated that the total expenditures of pharmaceutical companies in promoting their products to doctors was approximately $600 million in 1966—or about $3,000 per practicing physician—and about $900 million in 1968.[17] In 1971, promotional expenditures rose to about $1 billion. The Social Security Administration has charged that 85 percent of these expenditures "... must be classified as an economic waste." The agency further stated that:

Drug companies spend more promoting their drugs to doctors than they do on their highly publicized research, which cost slightly less than $700 million in 1971. The cost of promoting drugs to doctors also exceeds the

$977 million spent by the nation's medical schools during the academic year 1970–1971 to support all of their educational activities.[18]

Hospitalization

Nowhere is the physician less concerned with costs than he is in the hospital environment. In this environment, the physician can be expected to revert to the patterns of his medical school and specialty training periods. Here, only the highest quality medicine may be practiced. As a result, he is likely to care for his hospitalized patients with virtually no consideration for costs. Nursing care, laboratory tests and x-rays, special diets, physical therapy, and numerous other modalities, are often ordered with unwarranted frequency. This behavior by physicians is reinforced by peer pressure, since in no other setting does the physician's work receive as much scrutiny by other doctors as it does in the hospital setting.

Furthermore, although he may give some consideration to his patient's reaction to a bill for private office care, he is pleasantly relieved of this concern with the hospitalized patient. Often he knows, or assumes, that most costs will be borne by the insurance company and that he is free to practice the best and safest medicine that he knows.

The desire to practice in well-designed and well-equipped hospitals can also add to the financially irresponsible behavior of medical management. In this regard, physicians who sit on the boards of hospitals typically urge their fellow directors to build, expand, and overequip even though well-meaning federal subsidy programs have already created an oversupply of hospital facilities throughout the nation.

Hospital medical staffs, moreover, virtually always endorse purchases of items that will raise the hospital's equipment to the level of that in other hospitals. Thus, radiation treatment facilities, renal dialysis and intensive care units, tomographic scanners, and a large number of other costly services and equipment are purchased even when the community is already adequately supplied with such services and equipment in nearby hospitals.

The cost to society of additional facilities, services, and equipment, which is measured in spiralling costs for hospitalization, undoubtedly outweigh the benefits realized.

Laboratory Work

Many physicians order a greater number of laboratory tests than are indicated by their patients' conditions. In part they do so as a result of the fear of malpractice litigation—that is, the physician wants as complete a medical record as possible should he be required to defend himself in court. If he is sued, he will be required to demonstrate that he has provided the best possible health care. In some cases, moreover, esoteric tests may be conducted where they are not warranted simply to satisfy the intellectual curiosity of the physician. In the case of some physicians, each of these factors also serves to augment their earnings.

Physicians may purchase laboratory facilities and x-ray equipment and do their own diagnostic work rather than sending patients to outside laboratories and x-ray facilities. Thus, they earn the profits from diagnostic activities. Whereas the physician is ethically bound to give the best medical advice to his patients, anyone who sells a product at the same time that he offers advice related to that product experiences some conflict of interest. Unethical doctors have the opportunity to charge high fees for in-house laboratory work and x-rays, or even to order tests when none are needed, to generate income for themselves.

However, unethical doctors do not have to own laboratory equipment to earn income from the tests that they prescribe. An unethical physician can take a specimen in his office and, without the patient's knowledge, send it to an outside laboratory and charge the patient a fee that includes the laboratory cost, as well as an additional charge for himself. Some laboratories also have fee schedules that make this kind of physician behavior profitable, since they charge one fee if the laboratory takes the specimen and a lower fee if the physician takes it. For more expensive tests, which may consist of a number of tests performed simultaneously on automated equipment, the difference between the two rates can be great. As a result, the physician is encouraged to take his own specimens and keep the difference between the two rates for himself or to order expensive multiple tests rather than the less expensive and less profitable single test. Although some states have made such practices illegal, each new law only seems to create a number of alternative ways to continue the practice.

Unnecessary Surgeries

Many surgical procedures also fall into the area of overtreatment of patients. Most of these unrequired surgeries are performed in the fee-for-service environment rather than in prepaid practice. Indeed, a shocking proportion of the surgeries performed in the fee-for-service system appear to be unnecessary.

In a program sponsored by New York labor unions, all recommendations for surgery were required to be reviewed by a committee of independent board-certified specialists. The results of this program showed that 17.6 percent of the operations recommended by surgeons were found to be unnecessary by other surgeons who had no financial stake in the decision to operate.[19]

Other studies comparing surgery rates for federal employees covered by Blue Cross and by prepaid group practices showed remarkably different rates for the two. Assuming that the prepaid groups performed no excessive surgeries—an assumption considered to be conservative by those knowledgeable in the field—almost half of the Blue Cross surgeries would appear to have been unnecessary.[20]

Comparisons of rates of surgery in the United States and Great Britain indicate that Americans undergo twice as much surgery as do the British.[21] The assumption that the population of Great Britain receives at least an adequate amount of surgical procedures—which seems reasonable in view of the fact that medical care is readily available through the nation's sytem of national health care—suggests that about 50 percent of the surgeries performed in the United States would appear to be unnecessary. This differential is very close to that obtained during the three federal employee studies mentioned above.

The Social Security Administration conducted a carefully controlled study of comparable populations of Medicaid patients receiving care under prepaid health plans and fee-for-service.[22] It found that hospitalization was two and one-half times greater for patients cared for under fee-for-service than for members of prepaid group practices. The surgery rates for patients who were cared for under fee-for-service were double those for members of prepaid groups. Quality of care and characteristics of the Medicaid patients being compared were not explanations for the observed differences in hospitalization and surgery rates. Enrollment selectivity (previous health status), ambulatory-care use (including preventive care), accessibility, and patient satisfaction were remarkably similar in both prepaid and fee-for-service modes. Table 9-1 summarizes these studies.

Table 9-2 shows that if the present rates of surgery continue, the probability of an individual's having an operation by age seventy will be 45.3 percent for hysterectomy, 32.6 percent for inguinal hernia repair, and 30.1 percent for tonsillectomy. These rates for U.S. citizens are based almost entirely on experience under the fee-for-service system. By contrast, the probability of having such surgery is much lower in prepaid group practice.

Why is so much unnecessary surgery performed in the United States? Without a doubt, the fee-for-service incentive system is the primary cause. Under this payment mechanism, physicians earn more

Table 9-1. Unnecessary Surgery

Year	Population	% Unnecessary
1973	N. Y. Unions	17.6
1962	Federal Employees (Blue Cross vs. Prepaid Group)	44.3
1967	Federal Employees (Blue Cross vs. Prepaid Group)	53.5
1970	Federal Employees (Blue Cross vs. Prepaid Group)	46.2
1965	U. S. vs. England	49.0
1975	Medicaid Patients (Fee-for-Service vs. Prepaid Group)	50.0

Source: See endnotes 18 through 23 of this chapter.

Table 9-2. Probability of Having a Given Operation by Age 70.

Operation	U.S.	Prepaid Group
Hysterectomy	45.3%	16.8%
Primary Appendectomy	11.5%	7.0%
Tonsillectomy	30.1%	10.5%
Prostatectomy	17.5%	7.7%
Inguinal Herniorrhaphy (hernia repair)	32.6%	21.0%

Source: S. M. Wolfe, testimony in *Hearings* before the House Subcommittee on Oversight and Investigations on Unnecessary Surgery, Interstate and Foreign Commerce Committee, 94th Congress, 1st Session, Washington, D.C., July 15, 1975 (mimeo), p. 6.

money when they perform surgery than when they do not. Consider, for example, a patient suffering with a painful shoulder. If such a patient were a member of a prepaid group practice, he might be given injections and followed conservatively for as long as possible, perhaps even for years. If this same patient saw an orthopedic surgeon in the fee-for-service setting, however, the probability is much greater that he would receive surgery.

There are also other factors at work. Like all experts, surgeons want to apply the skills that they have devoted years to mastering. Moreover, unlike the more intellectual and methodical type of person who gravitates to internal medicine, the typical surgeon is a man of action who seeks definitive cures. Consequently, this aspect of the surgeon's personality increases the statistical likelihood of patients' receiving surgical treatment for any given illness. Moreover, this behavior is reinforced by the present oversupply of surgeons in the United States. Finally, since surgery is now safer than it once was, surgeons perform elective surgery more readily than they did in the past. Antibiotics can be used to fight infection, the quality of nursing care has improved, and life support systems reduce the danger of many surgical procedures. All of these factors reinforce the financial incentive of the surgeon to perform surgery whenever there is a borderline indication to do so.

Surgeons in well-conceived prepaid health plans, on the other hand, do not have a financial incentive to perform unnecessary surgery. Although they have the same behavior traits as fee-for-service surgeons, the financial incentives of prepayment help to restrain the impulse to perform unnecessary surgeries.

Surgeons in prepaid group practices have other opportunities for containing surgery rates, and these opportunities typically are not found in fee-for-service office based medical practices. First, the surgeon can consult readily with other surgeons in his group; they can allay his anxiety about cases. "Sit on it for awhile," they may advise him about a patient problem where there are borderline indications that surgery might be appropriate. Similarly, if a patient is demanding unnecessary surgery, other surgeons in the group can reinforce the advice that surgery is inappropriate. Advice from physicians in other specialties is also readily available, and the surgeon can consult with them without losing a fee through referral. The radiologist may be able to advise him that no biopsy is required for Mr. Johnston. The internist may be able to tell him that Mrs. Ambrose's problem is not what he worst suspected and that he will not need to make an abdominal incision to confirm his diagnosis. Finally, the prepaid plans employ fewer surgeons. Thus, any individual surgeon in a prepaid plan will perform more surgery than his fee-for-service counterpart. This provides a way for him to satisfy his desire to operate without the necessity of performing unnecessary surgery.

Sidney M. Wolfe, M.D., of the Public Citizen's Health Research Group, appeared before the House Subcommittee on Oversight and Investigations on July 15, 1975. He summarized studies indicating that 30 to 40 percent of hysterectomies are unnecessary.[23] This percentage translates into conservative estimates of 220,000 unnecessary hysterectomies a year, costing more than $330 million and resulting in 1,000 deaths. Wolfe further pointed out that, at present rates, 30 percent of the population will receive a tonsillectomy. Yet studies demonstrate that 50 to 75 percent of all tonsillectomies are unnecessary. Wolfe's estimates indicate, therefore, that 442,000 unnecessary tonsillectomies are performed each year at a cost of $331 million and the deaths of 100 children.

In 1973, 18.4 million operations were performed in the United States.[24] If 17.6 percent of these surgeries were unnecessary—a conservative view according to the studies summarized in Table 9-1— one can estimate that about 3.2 million unnecessary operations were performed, and a conservative average cost of $1,500 per surgery would mean that $4.8 billion per year is wasted in unnecessary surgery. When a conservative estimate of 0.5 percent mortality for elective surgery is taken into account, the needless loss of life amounts to 16,000 deaths per year.

If the 50 percent rate of unnecessary surgeries is used—the rate suggested by most studies—the cost in dollars and lives assumes an even greater magnitude. In this case, 9.2 million unnecessary surgeries are estimated to be performed each year at a cost of $13.8 billion and 46,000 lives—as many as the total number of Americans who lost their lives in the entire Vietnam War.

Whether these estimates ultimately prove to be too high or too low, the case seems compelling that a substantial amount of surgery performed in the United States is unnecessary.

Conclusions

Statistics on unnecessary surgery may represent only the tip of the iceberg. Because hospitals keep statistics on surgery, it is subject to some scrutiny, but this kind of scrutiny never reaches the individual physician's office. Yet the fee-for-service incentive rewards the physician for unnecessary medical care of all types. Although data are not available to support or refute the hypothesis, a reasonable expectation would be that the incidence of unnecessary nonsurgical care is at least as great as the rates of unnecessary surgery performed in hospitals.

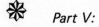 *Part V:*

Proposals for Reform

Chapter Ten

Proposals to Reform the Health Care System

Demands by social critics to reform the health care delivery system of the United States are the product of two fundamental criticisms. The first is a criticism of American health care itself. At its best, the quality of American medicine is the finest in the world. But it focuses too much on acute health problems and too little on keeping people well, too much on the ailments of the affluent classes and too little on the health problems of the poor. Consequently, access to health care is uneven.

The metropolitan physician generally spends many hours each week seeing middle-class patients, a large proportion of whom have no real need for a physician's attention. Because government will not reimburse physicians their UCR fees, the Medicaid patient is frequently turned away by the physician. The welfare patient consequently is forced to seek help at crowded county hospitals that may be located far from home. Too often children receive unnecessary tonsillectomies and women receive unneeded hysterectomies, while the medically isolated in some parts of rural and small-town America have no physicians at all. The quality of care is also open to criticism. Most physicians are very capable, but some would not be able to pass reasonable tests to certify their skills.

The second fundamental criticism of American medicine relates to its cost. The growth of health care expenditures is out of control, and the problem is becoming worse. The incentives implicit in public and private health insurance, the mismanagement of hospitals and physicians' offices, and the fee-for-service payment system all contribute to high and rising health care expenditures.

These criticisms are frequently made in an emotion-charged atmosphere. They produce angry charges and countercharges. In moments of calm, however, few would deny the truth of these criticisms, at least to a degree. The question over which people disagree primarily is what, if anything, should be done by government to improve health care delivery. Many suggestions have been made for reforming the delivery of health care services in the United States. These proposals, however, can be reduced to four main approaches: (1) nationalizing health care delivery; (2) extending national health insurance to the general population; (3) regulating the fee-for-service practice of medicine; and (4) promoting prepaid health plans to compete with the fee-for-service system of health care delivery.

Let us examine these alternatives.

NATIONALIZATION OF HEALTH CARE

Under a system of nationalized health care, facilities for the provision of health services would be owned and operated by the government, which would collect taxes to pay for the system. Individuals would be permitted to utilize the system as a matter of right, and no fees, or only nominal fees, would be collected at the time care was given to patients. Physicians and other health care providers would work for a salary.

The alleged merits of nationalization of health care are several. First, it would permit the government to assume responsibility for health care. Questions of how much should be spent on health care and of what kinds of health care services should be provided (e.g., preventive care versus acute care) would become social decisions made by the political process. Health policy would no longer be largely decentralized in the hands of individual physicians or hospitals. Under government control, decisions about how best to allocate health care resources could become matters of social policy, and as such would be less influenced than in fee-for-service health care by considerations of how physician earnings would be affected.

In pointing out the advantages of the accountability that would be gained by nationalization, Eveline M. Burns of Columbia University stresses that:

> . . . governmental participation in, or operation of, health services has two important advantages over private arrangements, namely, visibility and the existence of an authority that can be held responsible for shortcomings and has power to take remedial action. The most impressive feature of the British experience since 1948 has been the extent to which shortcomings

of the medical services as they affect the patient and the quality of care have been brought into the open and made the subject of public inquiry and remedial efforts.[1]

A second claim made for nationalization is that it would permit the government to reform the institutions that deliver care with a view toward improving their quality and efficiency. Burns notes that the "one truly revolutionary feature of the British Health Service was the possiblity offered, and taken, of restructuring the whole set of institutions so as to avoid wasteful deployment of resources."[2] The restructuring became necessary once the British taxpayer realized how extraordinarily costly the inefficient operations of the British hospital system had become.

Third, nationalization could help to reduce the uneven access to health care that now plagues the American health care system. Government could ensure that health care services were available throughout the country to all individuals, just as it now ensures that public schools are provided for all children.

However, nationalization of health care is not likely to be attempted in the United States in the near future. Whether it would ever be successful is also questionable. For one thing, physicians are adamant in their opposition to nationalized health care: They do not want to surrender their professional autonomy to the government; many also realize that nationalized medicine would eventually erode their earning power. Successfully imposing any health care reform on physicians over their strong opposition is thus unlikely. Moreover, a large segment of the public seems to be disinterested in nationalized health care. Rather, the politics of the 1970s seem to reflect a mood of skepticism about the ability of government to produce and manage social services with competence and efficiency.

The physicians and the public are probably right about the inadvisability of instituting nationalized health care in the United States. To do so would be to replace one set of management problems with another. Health care services are currently being produced inefficiently in the United States. Physicians are poor managers, and they face incentives that discourage the careful deployment of health care resources. But the record of government in organizing and managing social services in the United States is equally unimpressive. The post office and the welfare system, for example, are under attack by critics of all political persuasions. In all likelihood, then, government administrators will not prove to be better able to manage the day-to-day delivery of health care than are physicians.

Moreover, the ultimate outcome of nationalization could be that

the administration of health care services would continue to be controlled by physicians. William A. Glaser of Columbia University has
summarized this problem by pointing out that:

> ... even the most authoritarian decrees customarily contain some modifi-
> cations that would please the medical profession, since the government is
> anxious about any interruptions of medical service for which it will be
> blamed. Once agreements are made and doctors accept the system in
> practice, members of the profession are assigned to administer it, with the
> payment relegated to budgetary review. Therefore authoritarian and evolu-
> tionary solutions ultimately end at the same point. Elaborate concessions
> are made to the professions' demands for autonomy, resources, and incen-
> tives sufficient for future recruitment.[3]

Finally, the advantages offered by nationalization can be accomplished with less political upheaval by modest reform of the medical
incentives and management practices found in the present system.
Far too much is good about American health care delivery to justify
its total abandonment in favor of nationalized medicine.

NATIONAL HEALTH INSURANCE

Under a system of national health insurance, the government does
not produce health care services, as in nationalized health care, but
merely finances them. The financial details are handled in various
ways. Some countries place tax revenues in special trust funds and
pay the providers of health care from these funds. Others finance
health care out of general tax revenues. But, regardless of the institutional details, the purpose of national health insurance is to provide financial access to health services for all citizens.

In most of the developed countries, national health insurance is
well established for broad segments of the population. In the United
States, however, national health insurance has been limited to the
elderly, through Medicare, and to the poor, through Medicaid. Most
current proposals for extending national health insurance would provide coverage for catastrophic care to the entire population and
would extend full or comprehensive coverage only to people who are
considered to be in financial need and are not covered by Medicare
or Medicaid.

Reviewing all of the applicable bills now before the Congress is not
necessary here. Such reviews have already been made,[4] and most become obsolete rapidly as new bills are written and old ones are revised. But one thing is clear: Regardless of the form that national

health insurance might take, under the fee-for-service payment system physicians would submit bills to an administrative agency for all the services they deem necessary to provide for their eligible patients. The outcome would differ little from the country's experience under Medicare and Medicaid (as well as Blue Cross, Blue Shield, and private health insurance programs). An editorial in the *New York Times* expressed the matter well:

> An ironic element in [the] increase [in medical care costs] has been that every forward-looking reform for erasing the sometimes catastrophic burden of illness for low- and middle-income families—Medicare, Medicaid, and employer-financed insurance through Blue Cross and Blue Shield—has had the perverse effect of spurring the upsurge in overall costs.[5]

The reasons that costs rise with the advent of government and insurance health care programs are easy to understand. Health insurance, whether private or public, only provides purchasing power for the consumers of health care services. It does not change the incentives created by fee-for-service medical care.

The potential impact of national health insurance on the demand for health resources is enormous. In a Rand Corporation study published in 1974, Joseph Newhouse, Charles Phelps, and William Schwartz concluded that national health insurance could generate a 5 to 15 percent increase in demand for hospital care and a 30 to 75 percent increase in demand for ambulatory physician services. They also noted that "these represent conservative estimates of the changes that can be expected under each program."[6]

The American public should realize that fee-for-service medicine will prove to be a "black hole" capable of absorbing all the dollars they are willing to allocate to health care through national health insurance. The physician has a virtually endless number of services that he can provide. He can spend more time as physician counsellor, a fondly remembered role from the past. He can also turn his attention to other matters that he is fully qualified to handle: psychosomatic problems, diet and exercise counselling, control of alcohol consumption, emotional disturbance, child rearing and marriage counselling, and preventive medicine, to name only a few.

Walter McClure, a leading health analyst, makes the point well:

> ... the medical care system can legitimately absorb every dollar society will give it. If health insurance is expanded without seriously addressing the medical care system itself, cost escalation is likely to be severe and chronic. For example, why provide $50 of tests to be 95 percent certain of

a diagnosis if $250 of tests will provide 97 percent certainty. Or, if a patient's case looks hopeless, why not try an operation with a one-in-a-thousand chance of success if insurance will pay.[7]

Consider the economic impact of just one single surgical procedure that is now technically feasible in many parts of the country. The coronary artery bypass operation is considered by many physicians to be the preferred treatment for patients with disease of the coronary arteries (the vessels that supply blood to the heart itself). When blocked, the coronaries may cause heart pain known as angina pectoris. In some cases, this pain is relieved by a graft of leg vein to bypass the blocked coronary artery. However, not enough time has passed to tell whether there are any long-term benefits to be accrued from widespread coronary artery bypass surgery.

About four million people in the United States are known to have coronary artery disease. At least three million more are believed to have the disease. A further estimate is that there are about 700,000 new cases per year. In theory, about 85 percent of all patients with coronary artery disease are suitable for this operation because they have bypassable obstruction of their coronary arteries.

Duncan Neuhauser, a Harvard health economist, estimates that at today's typical rates for hospitalization, angiography (x-ray studies of the coronary arteries), and surgery, the cost to provide this procedure to the operable patients currently afflicted with coronary artery disease would be $46 billion.[8] This figure amounts to more than one-third the current annual health care expenditures in the United States. It is more than the annual expenditures for all public health, dental care, physician services, and medical research combined.

Coronary artery bypass surgery is only one item on a long list of therapeutic modalities that can find widespread application in health care if they are given sufficient funding. Like coronary artery bypass surgery, many of the most popular modalities are extraordinarily expensive, but may offer only marginal benefits. Kidney transplants could be made available to all patients meeting specified medical criteria. The federal government has recently considered creating kidney dialysis centers throughout the country to prolong the lives of patients with kidney disease. Technologic advances such as the tomographic "whole body" scanners will soon create a demand for preventive medical x-rays that visualize the body on cross-section so that we may all learn the degree of hardening of our arteries or the status of our vital organs, even though we are free of disease symptoms.

J. Enoch Powell, British Minister of Health over a decade ago, recognized that the health care system can prove to be a "black hole":

> Common thought and parlance tend to conceal or deny the fact that demand [for health services] for all practical purposes is unlimited. The vulgar assumption is that there is a definable amount of medical care "needed" and that if that "need" was met no more would be demanded. This is absurd.
> ... There is virtually no limit to the amount of medical care an individual is capable of absorbing.[9]

Despite its disadvantages, many political leaders and health planners continue to promote national health insurance, apparently unaware that the incentives in fee-for-service health care have created a system so seriously flawed that the simple addition of further consumer buying power may have disastrous economic effects. Typical of their attitude toward national health insurance is the following statement from a recent Department of Health, Education and Welfare publication:

> National health insurance (including the proper role of government) is probably the most crucial and compelling issue affecting the financing and cost of health care services, as well as the overall performance of our health care system. Past polarization has recently given way to broad agreement that the United States can and should adopt a system of health care financing that assures every person the opportunity to obtain necessary health care services at prices he or she can afford. Although specific proposals on how such a system could best be structured and administered, how costs should be distributed and contained, what degree and form of regulation would be called for, and what spectrum of benefits should be included, remain unresolved, we hope we are finally beyond the point of debating whether or not we will adopt a national health insurance system.[10]

Certainly a strong case can be made for a more equitable distribution of health insurance. A program that will ensure adequate access to care for the poor and for the near poor is needed. Coverage for catastrophic care is also highly desirable. But providing massive new expenditures for health care without simultaneously reforming health care incentives—and without simultaneously providing for adequate management of medical practices—will simply add more money to a system that has long demonstrated its inability to turn that money into new services that are efficiently produced. It is essential that reform precede national health insurance, for experience in other countries indicates that the institution of a national financing program tends to freeze evolution in the structure of the delivery system. National health insurance is advanced for noble reasons, but it will fail unless provision is also made to overhaul the current health care delivery system.

DIRECT REGULATION

Direct regulation of the health care industry has been attempted by the government, and self-regulation has been initiated by providers of health services—both in an attempt to control some of the most serious abuses found in the present health care delivery system. For example, the building of unnecessary hospitals in the United States is at least as scandalous an irresponsibility as the unnecessary surgery that is performed within them. A recent federal program established Comprehensive Health Planning Councils in virtually every community in the United States to review, among other things, hospital construction and equipment purchases. Since the government stopped short of giving the councils authority to block construction of even a small number of hospitals across the country, the program had little effect. The councils were even less effective in helping control the purchase of expensive hospital equipment and in promoting instead the cooperative use of such equipment among hospitals. The councils are now being phased out in favor of more powerful Health Systems Agencies, established by law under the National Health Planning and Resources Development Act of 1974. As yet, we cannot determine whether these new agencies will be any more effective than the Comprehensive Health Planning Councils in regulating the excesses of hospital boards and districts.

California's Secretary of Health and Welfare, Mario Obledo, has pointed out the ineffectiveness of the bureaucracies established by the Comprehensive Health Planning Councils. In a strongly worded attack, he argues that the government is making the same mistakes with the new Health Systems Agencies that it made with the Councils:

> Its efforts to date have focused on the development of a multitude of non-elected, super-government agencies, nominally in the hands of local regions, but, in effect, dependent upon not-yet-developed federal regulations and uncertain fiscal largess for survival. Two specific examples may illustrate the problem:

1. In California alone, approximately 400 persons (or a number ten times greater than our State Senate) will be appointed to various regional super-government Health Systems Agencies: These 400 persons may, in turn, be advised by sub-area groups of undetermined size and number. Further, these 400 unelected persons will participate in selecting a super-galactic health agency known as the Statewide Health Coordinating Council. These super-government Health Service Agencies will exist in tandem with 28 Medical Peer Service Review Organizations, 25 Councils of Government, 10 Councils of Inter-governmental Relations Planning Districts, and 58 duly-elected county governments, as well as the 165 duly-elected California state and federal legislators.

2. The Act will require these approximately 400 persons in California to hire professional staffs of at least 200 persons. One of the primary functions of these so-called experts will be to "complete initial review of existing institutional health services within three years after the date of the agencies' designations" despite the clear Congressional "urgency" clause and the health care crisis throughout the nation.[11]

Some states have tried to control health facility construction by passing certificate of need laws. These laws require that proposals for construction projects be submitted to a review board for approval prior to construction. Recognizing that local hospital administrators and physician staffs typically will support new construction, these laws usually provide for a large share of consumer representation on the review boards. An analysis of the effect of these laws leads to some disappointing findings: (1) projects usually are not reviewed within the context of a comprehensive plan; (2) because clear standards for determining need are seldom developed, nor are criteria established for measuring the financial feasibility of projects, decisions made in project reviews often appear to be arbitrary, (3) in many instances project review has increased construction costs by delaying projects while inflation has driven up prices; (4) giving the community a voice in the process tends to dilute efforts to contain capital expenditures, for members of the community are generally reluctant to vote against more or better health services, regardless of cost.[12]

Even if the Health Systems Agencies or some other form of direct regulation are able to provide effective regulation of hospitals—which is a doubtful proposition—such controls are unlikely to penetrate down to monitor abuses at the level of the individual physician's office. In fact, no federal, state, or local government has even attempted to control or monitor the physician's office practice. Government regulation, probably unavoidably, leaves the physician with total control over the location of his office, purchase of laboratory and x-ray equipment, and the services he provides his patients. Physicians also have full discretion over fees, although the government does attempt to set limits on the amount it will pay for health care procedures under its funded programs. (The effect, as has been noted, can be to undermine the willingness of physicians to participate in these programs.) Hence, direct regulation stands little chance of being able to monitor health care delivery in medical office practices.

The boards of medical examiners in every state exercise control over licensure of physicians. They suspend and revoke licenses of physicians because of alcoholism, drug abuse, and criminal activities. But even this regulation of blatant physician misconduct is not effective. For example, California's Board of Medical Examiners, which is the most active in the country, is currently under attack for not adequately policing physicians.

Estimates have been made, perhaps conservatively, that 5 percent of physicians in the United States are incompetent. These physicians see approximately 7.5 million patients each year for a total of 33.5 million visits. Seldom do boards of medical examiners revoke licenses for incompetence. In fact, in thirty-five of the states a physician's license cannot be challenged for professional incompetence.[13]

The Department of Health, Education and Welfare is currently sponsoring a new program to monitor the quality of care given by physicians in the hospital setting. Monitoring is accomplished through review by physician peers. Encouraged by a number of experiences in which county medical societies and hospitals have established successful peer review programs to police physician activities, the federal government, through its Professional Standards Review Organizations (PSROs), is trying to establish such programs across the country. But even if PSROs were to succeed—a questionable assumption given their tenuous acceptance by many physicians— there is little evidence that they could ever be able to extend their authority into the individual physician's office. Peer review programs are virtually always confined to hospital care, rather than to outpatient, private office care.

Overall, the potential for the long-term success of governmental regulation of health care is not bright. Even as the Health Systems Agencies have replaced the Comprehensive Health Planning Councils—only to be replaced in a few years by another governmental program with vague purpose, inadequate funding, and watered-down authority—physicians can expect that the Professional Standards and Review Organizations will be replaced by still other governmental experiments. One reason for this "musical chairs" approach of government to health care regulation is that all health programs share a common trait: They are the products of an unstable compromise between ideals and ideologies. As such, they are ineffectual, wasteful, and destined to be short lived.

George Pickett of the American Public Health Association addressed the problem of politics in national health policy by pointing out:

> Compromise, in American politics, has undergone a subtle change in process as we have moved from a confederation to a nation. The pork barrel has changed to a stew pot. Once upon a time a legislator with a particular goal could gain the votes needed by agreeing to support another legislator's goal in another unrelated bill. Laws were more regional and less national a century ago. But the process has become more national and more scientific. The author's desired objective is described accurately and then, through head counting, the contents of the bill are selectively modified to gain the number of votes needed. From inter-bill compromising we have shifted more towards intra-bill compromising. The process is, in some respects, faster, and our general societal acceleration has demanded this, but it is more difficult to find a clear sense of policy in the final law since the resulting bills reflect the ambivalence inherent in compromising values. The result is often left to administrative determination of national policy, which is less responsive to the electorate than the political process, and to occasional judicial surprises.[14]

Thus, a good idea that might become an effective reform is compromised and modified in the political process until it becomes unworkable.

A second reason is that the advocates of given health care regulations within government are political figures. Each official supports particular reform proposals. He helps push new regulations through Congress, and then typically he moves on to another job. When his programs run into difficulty, they are replaced by the new solutions of his successors.

The greatest weakness of direct regulation, however, lies not in the failure of regulation to have an effect, but in the likelihood that the regulation of medicine will come to serve the interests of physicians and other special interest groups rather than those of the general public. Such is the history of direct regulation. An economist's wry definition of a depressed industry is "one that has failed to capture its regulatory agency within five years after the agency is established." That is because appointments to regulatory agencies involve political considerations. As a result, seldom is an appointment made that is not satisfactory to those being regulated. In time, the regulators shift from their prescribed role and begin to see themselves as promoters of the industry that they are regulating. This shortcoming has been exhibited by the Interstate Commerce Commission, the Civil Aeronautics Board, the professional licensure boards of the states, and a myriad of other federal and state regulatory agencies.

HEALTH MAINTENANCE ORGANIZATIONS

The reform possibility with the greatest support among many health care planners is prepaid medical plans. The federal government is currently encouraging such reform by promoting the development of the Health Maintenance Organization (HMO). An HMO is a generic term referring to any medical plan that provides comprehensive care for its subscribers in exchange for a prepaid periodic payment. Under the Health Maintenance Organization Act of 1973, any employer with more than twenty-five employees who offers a health benefits plan must also give his employees the option of joining a federally qualified HMO if they live in an area served by such a prepaid health plan. The government hopes that this requirement will provide sufficient incentive for various organizations to establish HMOs and that many families will find them an attractive alternative to traditional health insurance and fee-for-service health care.

The 1973 HMO legislation provides for $375 million to be used by new HMOs for technical, feasibility, and planning studies. Advocates of HMOs anticipate that the cost of their health care services will be reasonable enough to make them attractive to large numbers of subscribers so that they will be able to provide competitive pressures to force some reorganization of fee-for-service health care delivery.

This legislation establishes two types of HMOs, "medical group" HMOs and "individual practice association" HMOs. The former is modeled on prepaid group practice plans such as that of Kaiser. The latter is based on the medical foundation. Medical foundations are decentralized health plans, originally established in California by county medical societies in an attempt to meet the competition of Kaiser. These foundations negotiate with representatives of a group of health care consumers—for example, a union—and agree to provide health care for members of that group in return for a prepaid capitation. In some of these plans, the foundation is "at risk" but not the individual physician who merely sees patients and is reimbursed by the foundation at predetermined fees. Such foundations differ little in economic impact from fee-for-service health care, because the physician's income depends directly on the volume of services he provides. Their costs per patient, hospitalization utilization, and surgery rates differ little from those of fee-for-service health care.[15] In well-conceived independent practice association HMOs, however, the physicians in the plan are "at risk"—that is, they agree to accept a capitation, and the difference between that revenue and the cost of care is theirs to keep. Incentives in such groups are quite conducive to cost containment and good management.

The growth of prepaid health plans has been slower than their advocates had hoped. Although more than five million enrollees are already receiving health care in more than one hundred prepaid plans, only a few plans have become certified as federally qualified HMOs under the 1973 Act.[16] Confusion about the requirements for a group practice to qualify as an HMO under the act has slowed the development of these plans. Furthermore, a few prepaid health plans have been formed by unscrupulous doctors and businessmen who have collected capitations and subsequently have provided substandard medical care. A number of the new plans have already gone bankrupt.

In concept, the HMO is sound. If the programs succeed, the problem of inadequate access to health care in some parts of the nation should be alleviated. Since prepayment is a cornerstone of HMOs, the fee-for-service incentive that has created so many problems is eliminated. Physicians generally are "at risk" or work for a salary and have no incentive to overtreat patients or to provide other unnecessary care, such as hospitalization,when outpatient care is sufficient. HMOs also could easily be combined with national health insurance, should the public decide that it wants to increase governmental financing of health care services. Most important of all, HMOs could provide a competitive alternative to the fee-for-service sector of health care delivery.

The response of some physicians who oppose HMOs is to protect their autonomy under the fee-for-service system by defending "freedom of choice" and the "doctor-patient relationship" and to play a waiting game by simply standing by in the hope that HMOs will collapse of their own weight. These physicians correctly perceive that government-sponsored change, particularly an elimination of fee-for-service health care, must come slowly, if at all. And it must come in a system that will be acceptable to the physicians.

Despite physician resistance, many of the problems incurred in initiating HMOs have resulted not so much from an unwillingness of physicians to practice prepaid health care, as from their frustrations in dealing with government. The federal government has been slow in defining the criteria it will use for certifying HMOs for federal qualification. Many doctors believe that even after their publication, the rules will be amended and revised repeatedly. Funding to implement the 1973 law, moreover, has been uncertain as organized medicine lobbies with the White house to shut down federal support for HMOs. Some physicians also see some danger in giving up their style of medical practice to accommodate the HMOs only to see the federal government eventually shift its attention and support to another approach.

In the final analysis, HMOs have suffered from two serious problems. First, many of them have been poorly managed. Yet good management is both difficult and crucial to an HMO's success. This is partly because prepayment makes medical care a right for subscribers by eliminating or virtually eliminating user fees for service. A prepaid plan must therefore find efficient ways of keeping up with the influx of patients which that right can produce.[17] Moreover, it is very difficult to predict the costs for a new prepaid health plan. Consequently, some HMOs, uncertain of costs but eager to find subscribers, committed themselves to subscriber rates that were too low to pay for quality health care services.

State laws, which had the effect until quite recently of making the legal status of HMOs ambiguous, contributed to their management problem. Until new laws were passed in a number of states, competent nonphysician managers, particularly business corporations, encountered difficulties in seriously considering organizing an HMO.

The second serious problem faced by HMOs was a direct consequence of the 1973 HMO Act itself. The Act required qualifying HMOs to offer a broad range of services, including not only hospitalization, the services of physicians, laboratory and other diagnostic services, and emergency care, but also mental health care, preventive dental care for children, home health services, and care for drug and alcohol abuse. In addition, federally qualifying HMOs were required to charge all subscribers a uniform "community rate," although insurance companies are permitted to charge higher rates for higher-risk groups of health care consumers. The act also required qualifying HMOs to allow "open enrollment" of individuals every year regardless of their health. The net result was that the HMO was effectively priced out of the market for many if not most health care consumers. HMOs had the option, of course, of not trying to qualify under the 1973 HMO Act, but if they followed this course of action they also had to forgo the "dual option" clause of the act that required employers to make a qualified HMO available to their employees. In addition, they could not obtain any of the federal loans provided by the act.

As Paul Starr, a Harvard University fellow, has put it:

> The fundamental problem with the law, however, was that it took no account of historical or economic realities. It asked that emerging HMO's undertake at the outset all the services that the most comprehensive plans provide after years of development. It made no allowances for the kind of normal evolution that successful plans have historically undergone. It placed requirements on HMO's that do not apply to their competitors and that prejudice their chances of survival. It ignored the limited purchasing power available for health services, particularly among lower-income groups. In sum, it made most difficult the form of organization it was ostensibly designed to promote.[18]

By mid-1976, amendments were before the Congress to correct many of the problems of the 1973 HMO Act. But as Starr has noted, the problems created by the 1973 law "may be alleviated by legislative amendments but they will not disappear: The structure of the program has been set, and much damage already done."[19]

In Summary

The four proposals for reforming the health care industry discussed in this chapter—nationalization, national health insurance, direct regulation, and the HMO—all share the basic problem that has been the subject of this book. All of them fail to provide, in one way or another, for efficient and effective management of health care delivery.

Nationalization of the health care industry would replace the physicians' poor management with management by government bureaucracy. Government's record in managing and producing social services in the United States is not impressive. True, nationalization would eliminate some of the problems of physician incentives by abolishing or strictly limiting the practice of fee-for-service medicine. But nationalization is no cure for the problem of physician incentives. In virtually all countries that have attempted extensive governmental management of health care, significant concessions have had to be made to permit fee-for-service reimbursement so that adequate quantities of professional services would be available.

To the extent that the second proposal, national health insurance, is viewed as a sufficient reform for American medicine, it will fail because it ignores the issue of incentives. Adding national health insurance to the nation's hospital-oriented medicine, practiced by office-based physicians utilizing the fee-for-service system, will merely increase the money spent on health care in the United States. It will not enhance the nation's ability to produce health care services effectively or efficiently. As has happened with Blue Cross and Blue Shield, and later with Medicare and Medicaid, the soaring health costs brought about by infusions of new purchasing power will soon lead to reductions in the eligibility of those served by the system and to cutbacks in the care promised patients. National health insurance is certainly justified on the grounds that adequate health care must be provided for all segments of society. But to be successful, it must be accompanied by reform of incentives.

One would be naive to anticipate that direct regulation can be successful in reforming the present system of health care delivery. The political process is not effective in designing or administering viable regulations. Successful regulation would require cooperation by the country's physicians. It would also need to avoid becoming an instrument that promotes physicians' special interests instead of the larger public interest. But there are few encouraging signs that either of these requirements can be met and sustained.

Prepaid medical practice—the HMO concept—currently offers the best hope for reform of health care delivery. First, it deals directly with the problems raised by the fee-for-service incentive. It solves these problems because physicians in prepaid HMOs are "at risk" or work on salary and have no financial incentive to provide unnecessary care for their patients. Second, to succeed, prepaid practice does not require the active support of even a majority of physicians. If such plans prove attractive to patients and to even some physicians, they will grow and prosper. If they offer care that is perceived to be superior to that given in traditional fee-for-service office-based practices, clinics, and hospitals, and if their costs are lower than those of mainstream medicine, then mainstream practice would be forced to change or gradually to convert to prepaid practice.

But the federal HMO legislation is an example of a good concept badly executed. To qualify under the law, an HMO must submit to too much regulation and provide a noneconomic health plan to consumers. To bypass qualification is to give up the advantages of "dual option" and attractive federal loans. It is not a good choice to have to make, and the dilemma provides a poor incentive for the advancement of the HMO concept.

TRANSFORMING PHYSICANS
INTO MANAGERS

One approach to solving the problems of medical management discussed in this book might be to train physicians to become effective managers. But this solution, although logical, is both impractical and impossible. Premedical students and medical students are already required to undertake years of difficult training and have little room in their schedules for additional required courses. Moreover, changing the medical school curricula is difficult to accomplish. Most important, even if training in business were made available to medical students, there is little reason to expect that physicians could become good managers merely by attending a small number of college courses. On-the-job training is also impractical because the demands on the physician's time are so great that he has little time for learning how to be a manager.

The physician's first concern is the care of his patients. His greatest social value, moreover, is in the practice of medicine. To involve him extensively in business management is to waste a highly expensive, specialized social asset. In addition, most doctors do not like being managers. Many people believe in a myth that physicians are rugged, entrepreneurial people who would be unable to function in a world where they were supervised by others. Many physicians believe this myth about themselves. But the truth is just the opposite. Many, perhaps most, physicians would gladly give up their responsibilities as business managers—if they could continue to earn as much as they now earn and expect to earn in the future and if they could maintain professional autonomy in medical decisions. Sufficiently compensated and given a choice to provide quality medicine, physicians would work outside the private, fee-for-service office setting. They defend the fee-for-service payment system mainly because they expect that their incomes and their medical autonomy will be eroded if they depart from the present system.

The physician as a manager, even with training, is not the answer to the problems of medical management. Physicians like to practice medicine, and they will serve society best if they concentrate on helping their patients rather than engaging in business and management. Any system that is to successfully reform health care delivery in the United States must pay special attention to this fact.

Chapter Eleven

The Corporate Practice
of Medicine

Given the drama that surrounds attempting to reform the health care delivery system by some combination of nationalization, national health insurance, regulation, and the Health Maintenance Organization, perhaps not surprisingly, little attention has been paid to another reform possibility of considerable potential significance. This approach is the practice of medicine by business corporations. Business corporations have been practicing medicine in one form or another for at least forty years, and in the last few years they have begun to find new ways to penetrate the health care sector. Although the activity of business corporations in the practice of medicine to date is hardly of revolutionary proportions, their entry into health care could ultimately prove to be more important than any other reform proposal for controlling costs and preventing unnecessary care.

Although business corporations have practiced medicine for many years, until recently they have done so in a fairly limited set of circumstances. Many corporations, for example, employ physicians and other medical personnel who care for the company's employees during working hours. The objective of these companies is to keep their labor force on the job. Large numbers of business corporations also practice preventive medicine by hiring doctors to give physical examinations. Often these are pre-employment physicals, but sometimes they are given to existing employees and are accompanied by counselling for weight control, alcohol abuse, exercise programs, and the like. Commonly hospitals, both non-profit and proprietary, have employed radiologists, pathologists, and a variety of consulting phy-

sicians, though this practice has been made difficult by legal problems. Kaiser Industries pioneered in prepaid health care with the
famed Kaiser Health Plan, established first for Kaiser employees and
their families, and later for other health care consumers. In recent
years, some groups of business investors and physicians have found
ways to go into business together to practice fee-for-service medicine;
typically, the nonphysicians operate within a profit or nonprofit
corporation and contract with the physicians who are members of a
professional corporation, thus eluding state laws that prohibit nonphysicians from employing doctors.

Passage of the Health Maintenance Act of 1973 stimulated a number of business corporations to consider forming HMOs. Some have
already done so. But most corporations evidencing early interest
were discouraged by the recession of the early 1970s that dried up
their venture capital, by the restrictive provisions of the 1973 Act itself, and by legal uncertainties about state restrictions and about malpractice vulnerability they might face. Since 1973, however, HMO
enabling legislation in a majority of states, plus attempts by the
federal government to reform the 1973 HMO Act to make federal
qualification more attractive, have improved the climate for business
investors and corporations interested in organizing HMOs.

The outlook is now better than it has ever been for business corporations to enter the health care field. Some could follow the
Kaiser model and start prepaid plans for the families of their employees. The soaring costs of company health care packages now
being offered through the mainstream fee-for-service sector could
provide the incentive for business corporations to try to gain control
of health care costs while offering their employees a well managed,
cost effective prepaid health plan. Like the Kaiser plan, some of
these health care plans could be expected to evolve into programs for
nonemployee groups as well. Still other business corporations could
form prepaid health plans as business investments and market them
to nonemployee groups at the outset.

Business corporations that entered the health care system with
prepaid health plans might also consider moving into fee-for-service
practice as well. A business corporation operating a prepaid health
plan would inevitably be asked to care for injured people in its emergency room. It would be acting irresponsibly if it did not find some
way to provide the necessary care and might reasonably be expected
to bill the patient on a fee-for-service basis. Should the corporation's
prepaid plan possess specialized services not found elsewhere in the
community, for example, a cancer treatment center or a highly

specialized eye surgeon, the community would have every right to expect the plan to accept fee-for-service patients on referral. From these beginnings, then, business corporations might gradually penetrate the full fee-for-service medical market.

Although some legal resistance would be expected as business corporations enter fee-for-service medicine, it is not at all clear that the law could be used effectively to prevent determined business investors. Medical societies attempted to use state licensure laws to block the establishment of prepaid group practice by Kaiser and others, but ultimately failed in a number of legal tests in the courts. Hospitals hired physicians, either directly or by contracting for them through professional corporations, even though the letter of the law in many states made such practice illegal.

Corporate practice of medicine in the HMO setting has a number of clear social advantages. The HMO would be subject to the incentives inherent in prepaid health care: to control costs and to avoid unnecessary care. Equally important, corporate HMOs would have the advantage of competent management and adequate financing, qualities missing in a number of existing HMOs.

The social implications of business corporations' practicing medicine in the fee-for-service sector are more problematical. A natural worry is that business investors would "control" their physicians in the interest of profit and, in the process, harm the patient. Another unclear area is how the problem of incentives for unnecessary care would be improved if nonphysician investors were to establish themselves to a significant degree in fee-for-service health care. An effective case can be made, however, that society would be no worse off with business corporations in the fee-for-service sector than it is now, and it might be better off. Already many physicians allow financial considerations to influence them to provide unnecessary care. Business investors, concerned about the reputations of their companies, might actually be less inclined than physicians to offer unnecessary care. Most important, society could be certain that business corporations would produce medical services more efficiently and effectively than they are produced today by physician businessmen.

As in the past, an important consideration for business corporations contemplating entry into medical practice is the formidable legal obstacles that have been erected by the states. These obstacles have been lowered somewhat by the 1973 HMO Act and by HMO enabling legislation in a majority of the states. Examining the legal barriers that have existed in the past will help in understanding the current legal environment.

A HISTORY OF LEGAL RESTRICTIONS TO
THE CORPORATE PRACTICE OF MEDICINE

By law, the practice of medicine has been limited to physicians. This restriction has been strengthened in all states by licensure laws enforced by physician-dominated state boards of medical examiners. The licensure stipulations are contained in the medical practice acts of the various states. Most of these acts stipulate that only physicians may engage in the practice of medicine and that all of those engaging in this practice must be licensed by the state. Some states expressly forbid for-profit organizations to participate in the provision of health care services.

The logic behind these laws is clear. Physicians are to be trusted in the financial aspects of medical care, but nonphysicians are considered to be interested primarily in profit rather than in the welfare of the patient. Thus, participation in health care by for-profit business corporate entities has been considered suspect.

Claims have been made that (1) consumers of health services are ignorant about medicine, (2) laws restricting entry into medicine are necessary to protect the unwary from incompetent medical practitioners, and (3) corporations owned and operated by anyone other than physicians would commercialize the profession and by so doing might harm innocent patients. Inherent in such logic has been a belief that the medical profession regulates its own quality with reasonable effectiveness. Hence, the public should be protected from the activities of persons and organizations not licensed and regulated by the profession.

The most common argument, then, against the entry of nonmedical personnel has been that nonphysician interference with the practice of medicine gives rise to divided loyalties on the part of the physician, who might be influenced by his corporate employer to consider factors other than the well-being of the patient. Specifically, the concern exhibited by such legislation has been that a corporation will influence a physician to place profit for himself and for the corporation above other considerations in patient care.

Regardless of the rationale claimed by the courts—and on occasion by legislatures and state attorney generals—the result of prohibitions on the corporate practice of medicine is restraint of trade. By limiting the practice of medicine to licensed physicians and then by restricting the possibilities under which physicians may be allowed to practice medicine, competition is reduced. As a consequence, traditional fee-for-service, office-based practice has been made more profitable for physicians than it would have been if they had had to face efficiently managed business corporations that employed physicians.

Clark C. Havighurst, Professor of Law at Duke University, has criticized some of the usual justifications for restrictive licensure:

> It is ironic that ethics and the quality of care have been so successfully advanced as justifications for restrictive legislation and professionally authorized restraints of trade. Whether this was always wholly a pretext on the part of the proponents of restrictive policies is of course doubtful, but the total effect was a raising of the cost of care and the incomes of health professionals. It was apparently not recognized that the allegedly high ethical and quality standards resulting from these exclusionary practices would be heavily paid for, not only in cash by paying patients but also in the suffering and lives of those who were effectively denied care.[1]

In his 1970 proposal to make the health care industry a market-oriented system, Havighurst further observed that:

> A combination of "ethics," customs of trade, and pressures of varying degrees of subtlety have repressed even the vestiges of price competition in the delivery of physicians' services. Under these conditions, the market has never had a chance. It is thus ironic in a purportedly free-enterprise system that, where radical reforms of the health care delivery system are being proposed on every side, the most radical reform possible might be restoration of a free market.[2]

Exclusive licensure was used for years to hinder the growth of prepaid health plans, such as Kaiser and the Health Insurance Plan of New York, until law suits in a number of states forced a relaxation of the legal interpretations. One should note that the only form of group practice opposed by medical organizations was prepaid group practice. The aim was to keep this new form of competition out of medicine. Physicians appear to have been more concerned about the impact of prepaid group practice on their incomes than they were about possible impacts on the quality of care. And laws that forbade business corporations from operating medical practices have reflected this same concern.

Without laws to restrain competition in medicine, new practice modes, including a variety of HMOs, might have developed much sooner. Rosemary Stevens, in *American Medicine and the Public Interest*, has postulated that:

> Had the medical profession not been a "profession," that is, if its members had been free to set up combinations of skills and types of personnel,

without the formal restraints of licensing laws and medical ethics and the informal restraints of guild fraternalism, the most congenial American pattern for organizing health services would almost certainly have been independent, voluntary associations of specialists and other health personnel, organized on efficient business lines and offering a clearly specified range of services. As an inducement, such organizations could have offered prepayment, extended payment and credit plans. In this event, health insurance plans (at least for the middle class working population) would be organized on a local basis, as illustrated in the handful of significant prepaid group practices which did develop in the United States.[3]

In his analysis of restraint of trade in medicine, the economist Milton Friedman has suggested:

Group practice and prepaid medical plans may have good features and bad features, but they are technologic innovations that people ought to be free to try out if they wish. There is no basis for saying conclusively that the optimum technical method of organizing medical practice is practice by an independent physician. Maybe it is group practice, maybe it is by corporations. One ought to have a system under which all varieties can be tried.[4]

Surprisingly, few business corporations or consumer groups challenged the laws banning the corporate practice of medicine. Most of the criticism of these laws has come from hospitals, both proprietary and nonprofit. These hospitals, however, have not been primarily concerned with adding competition and efficient business management to the health care field, but rather with legitimizing the arrangements by which hospitals employ or contract with physicians. A New York City Commissioner of Hospitals, reacting to the decisions limiting the corporate practice of medicine made by a number of courts in the 1930s, stated:

If the employment of a physician by a hospital for any medical purpose is the practice of medicine by the hospital, the Federal Government, every state in the Union, many hundreds of cities and counties, state and private universities, ecclesiastical hospitals of many denominations, and non-sectarian community hospitals, are engaged in the practice of medicine.[5]

By 1960, state attorney generals had divided on the issue, giving rise to concern that the very existence of public and community hospitals was being threatened. Virtually all hospitals retain the services of a pathologist to supervise the hospital laboratory and to perform surgical tissue studies and autopsies. They also employ radiologists to interpret x-ray studies. Both pathologists and radiologists, and a number of other consultant physicians, are still the center of a debate as to the legality of hospitals' practicing medicine through their physician employees.

Alanson W. Willcox, General Counsel of the American Hospital Association, observed in 1960:

> In dealing with the corporate practice of medicine we are faced by two facts which are exceedingly difficult to reconcile. The first is that courts have said over and over again that the corporate practice of medicine, dentistry and the like is illegal. The second is that, with the knowledge and acquiescence of all concerned, there are corporations in every state of the Union which are hiring physicians to practice medicine and which are furnishing, through physicians, a considerable portion of the medical care of the American people. . . .
>
> One is warranted in casting a skeptical eye at the statement of a rule of law in such broad terms as seemingly to condemn practices which are all but universally accepted tacitly if not explicitly, both in hospitals throughout the Nation and in large segments of the organization of medical care outside of hospitals. No one supposes that the rule would be applied to all these practices, despite the breadth of its usual statement, and distinctions have been suggested as means of keeping the rule within bounds. Most of these distinctions have as yet received little or no overt judicial support, but there are a great many decisions that either turn a blind eye to the corporate practice rule or decline to apply it on grounds which, if consistently applied, would go far toward reducing the rule to a nullity. There are signs that the courts themselves are troubled by the broad sweep of the rule as they have generally pronounced it.[6]

Fears of commercialization account for the hard stand taken by the earlier courts regarding the corporate practice of medicine. The legal literature is replete with examples of concern that for-profit corporations would more likely "control professional acts and professional judgments" than would nonprofit corporations. In this regard, the Attorney General of Minnesota advised:

> The distinction made by the cases between business corporations and nonprofit corporations is based upon sound considerations of public policy and persuasive reasoning. The objectionable features of the "corporate practice of medicine," or of any other profession, as stated by the Minnesota Supreme Court in the cases cited above, and by the numerous other courts that have considered the problem, are that the exploitation of the profession leads to abuses and that the employment of the doctor by a business corporation interposes a middleman between the doctor and the patient and interferes with the professional responsibility of the doctor to the patient. The corporation considered here would be nonprofit and

has a provision in the articles of incorporation prohibiting the corporation from intervening in the professional relationship between the doctors and the member-patients and confining the corporate activities to the economic aspects of medical and dental care. Therefore, a corporation so organized would not be subject to the objections urged against the business corporations that have been held prohibited from entering this field.

It is, accordingly, my opinion that a corporation organized as a nonprofit corporation for the purpose of carrying on the activities referred to in the statement of facts above is organized for a "lawful purpose," and, therefore, may be incorporated under the Minnesota Nonprofit Corporation Act.[7]

The long-term result has been the establishment of a number of nonprofit corporations whose sole reason for being is to engage in the practice of medicine. How they would do this any differently if they were for-profit corporations is difficult to imagine. Certainly they are as interested in profit as any other business. Perhaps the problem results from the connotations implied by the word "profit" as interpreted by those distrustful of the free enterprise system and the American business community.

The debate, then, over what constitutes the illegal corporate practice of medicine has led to a number of legal opinions and interpretations. The courts have been most sensitive to the issue of the "control" of medical practice. Any agreement or contract between a corporation and a physician that might influence the way in which the physician practices medicine is to be avoided. Consequently the courts have traditionally taken issue with any loss of physician independence. Thus, the contracts of hospital physicians who receive a share of the revenue generated by their medical services were readily and repeatedly attacked. The courts contended that the power to hire and discharge and to fix the compensation of an employee physician necessarily implies the power to control his work. Hospitals that established the fees for a physician's services and took control of the collection or receipt of such fees invited trouble in almost all states.

In attacking this view, the American Hospital Association argued:

The essence of all legitimate medical practice is a direct dealing between the individual physician and his patient, and this is no less true because payment may be routed to or through a corporation. There is no reason that a corporation may not contract to provide the services of a third person and receive payment therefore, without making the acts of that person its acts.[8]

A typical court opinion, however, stated:

> Professions are not open to commercial exploitation as it is said to be
> against public policy to permit a "middleman" to intervene for profit in
> establishing the professional relationships between the members of said
> profession and the members of the public.[9]

In 1972, the Attorney General of California gave an opinion that a
physician's percentage contract with a hospital indicated that the
physician's practice was not wholly owned and entirely controlled by
him within the meaning of the state's Business and Professions Code.
The general counsel for the California Hospital Association responded with understandable dismay:

> The opinion issued by your office questions the legality of what may be
> characterized as the typical type of arrangement that exists between hospi-
> tals and physician specialists performing services in the hospital. The effect
> of this opinion, if ultimately upheld by the courts, would be to destroy
> long-standing and mutually acceptable arrangements between hospitals
> and physician specialists in over 90 percent of the hospitals operating with-
> in this state. The impact on the health care system would be tremendous
> and alternatives to the existing procedures are difficult, costly and prejudi-
> cial to the interests of patients, hospitals, and medicine, as well as the
> state. The adverse effect on both quality of care and cost of care is incal-
> culable.[10]

The fact that noncompliance with the letter of the law has been
almost universal hardly encouraged American industry to pioneer in
the field of health care services. Most likely, the fear of being one of
the first major test cases to receive scrutiny by a board of medical
examiners helps explain the wait-and-see attitude of private industry.

Changes in the Law

With the Health Maintenance Organization Act of 1973 came
some relaxation in restrictive laws that had been used in the past to
limit the growth of prepaid health plans. The 1973 Act declared that
if a federally qualified HMO was prohibited from practicing in a state
because the state's law required approval of the HMO by the state
medical society; if state law required the HMO to be physician
dominated; if state law required an HMO to open participation to all
physicians or nearly all physicians in the geographic area to be served
by the HMO; or if state law required the HMO to meet special insurance requirements, then the state law would not apply. The 1973 Act

also declared that states may not prohibit solicitation of subscriber patients by an HMO.

Even with this superseding of state law, the laws of many states continued to make it difficult to establish HMOs. The Conference Board warned in a 1974 report entitled *Industry Roles in Health Care* that the private sector would be unable to bring its financial and managerial resources into the health care field until new enabling federal legislation was passed. The report added:

> The legal status of HMO's has been ambiguous, and it differs from one state to the next. Estimates of the number of states that would prohibit some form of HMO range from 22 to 49. It is doubtful that many more than a few would allow the creation of for-profit groups.[11]

But persuaded that HMOs deserve a chance to compete with fee-for-service practice, state legislatures began to enact HMO enabling laws. By midyear 1976 more than half the states had enacted such laws. Although other states have remained silent, some have given tacit approval to their formation.

The result of this new legislation is that the possiblity now exists for business corporations to organize and manage HMOs. In a majority of states, business corporations can establish HMOs in straightforward fashion. In every state, moreover, a business corporation could get itself licensed as an insurance carrier and use the carrier as a vehicle for forming an HMO. (Forming an HMO in this way can be quite expensive, however, as the HMO is required to meet the financial criteria applied by state law to insurance carriers.)

State laws vary as to whether a business corporation can operate a for-profit HMO or whether it must form a nonprofit corporation. In approximately twenty of the states, legislation is sufficiently flexible to permit business corporations to operate for-profit HMOs. However, investors in HMOs are at some disadvantage if they are required to establish nonprofit HMOs. Nonprofit HMOs cannot legally distribute dividends to shareholders, since by definition they have no profits to distribute. Moreover, if the corporation seeks tax exemption under the federal laws, it may face even more restrictions. Hence, business investors in a nonprofit HMO may encounter difficulties in getting their money out of the firm. Their only ways of doing so are through salaries and as payment for services performed. One avenue open to them, however, is to offer a service to the HMO—for example, a business systems procedure or some administrative services—and to take income from the HMO by performing the service. Although these restrictions pose no particular problem for HMOs organized by groups of physicians (who can take money

out of the HMO in the form of salary to themselves), a requirement that an HMO operate with nonprofit status could lessen
the attractiveness of HMOs as an investment for business corporations.

Those states that permit for-profit HMOs are more fertile ground
for business corporations. Even in these states, however, state law
still controls medical licensure and specifies whether or not corporations may practice medicine by directly employing physicians in
their HMOs. Although these laws do not erect insurmountable
barriers to business corporations, they do necessitate that investors
contemplating establishing an HMO seek competent legal advice.

One of the most important competitive advantages that business
corporations have in forming HMOs is the opportunity to bring
efficient management to health care delivery. In states where physicians can legally be employees, investors can attempt to establish
competent management by providing it themselves. But only a few
states permit physicians to be employees. In most states. business
corporations must contract with physicians through professional corporations of doctors. These are corporations limited to physician
shareholders. They are monitored closely by state boards of medical examiners. Careful attention must be given, then, to finding ways
to promote efficient management within the professional corporation short of violating prohibitions against the corporate practice of
medicine.

A perfectly legal practice, one should note, is for a group of investors to negotiate with a group of doctors an agreement under
which the professional corporation has strong incentives for good
management. Placing the professional corporation "at risk" by requiring it to operate solely on the income it derives from prepaid
capitations, rather than having each doctor operate strictly on a
salary with no incentives for hard work, is one such approach. The
nonphysician investors and the physicians can also agree to establish
peer review by the physicians to control unnecessary surgery and
hospitalization, and they can agree to provide for a competent business manager with adequate authority to make sure that office procedures are carried out efficiently and effectively.

Any business corporation contemplating forming an HMO, then,
must start by locating competent legal advice. Corporation execu-
tives need help in determing whether the law permits formation of a
for-profit HMO in any given state, in deciding whether to seek federal qualification under the 1973 HMO Act initially or whether to
organize with eventual qualification as a goal, in finding ways to
assure that the HMO will be operated efficiently without illegally
interfering with physician care of patients, and so forth. Finding such

legal advice is not easy. Few attorneys know about the current status of the law. Estimates have been made that in many states there is not a single legal firm that understands health law enough to provide up-to-date advice on establishing an HMO. A small number of specialized law practices do exist, however; these tend to have a national practice. Often, a sensible strategy for a business corporation is to retain local counsel and then to utilize a specialized firm as referral counsel.

CORPORATE ENTRY INTO THE HEALTH CARE SYSTEM

In the past, despite the problems that have confronted them, some for-profit corporations have been active in health-related industries. The most notable example was in the clinical laboratory business. Smith, Kline & French, Upjohn, Bristol-Myers, and a number of other drug manufacturers seeking diversification opportunities in the 1960s purchased medical laboratories to provide physicians with services with low costs that would reflect volume production, state-of-the-art automated analysis equipment, and the efficient business management of established corporations in the health field. Their hope was that they could sell laboratory services to physicians in a manner similar to the way they market drugs. What these firms failed to realize, however, was that physicians can own and operate laboratories or invest in them so that they can profit from referring their patients' laboratory work to their own laboratories. The problem of physicians' incentives taught the drug giants a bitter lesson about the medical industry. Few remain in the medical laboratory business today.

Likewise, a number of corporations have attempted to offer management talent and business efficiency to the hospital industry. Some companies that offer management service contracts to hospitals have been quite profitable. However, companies that have attempted to enter the hospital business itself have learned that the nation has far too many hospitals. Although hospitals are reimbursed by government funds, they also are increasingly coming under the profound influence of government rules and controls. Indeed, many people believe that the entire hospital industry will become a public utility within the next ten years. This unsettled state makes the investment of private capital quite speculative.

Both of these examples should serve as a warning that establishing HMOs may also involve special problems, even though many of the legal impediments to entry into the industry have been eliminated.

One problem is the chaotic status of medical malpractice litigation. An American Hospital Association monograph points out:

> A court may hold a corporation not guilty of corporate practice of medicine in the absence of lay control of the physician or lay intervention between him and his patient, and yet on a very similar state of facts hold the corporation liable for a tort committed by the physician.[12]

A number of business corporations have considered establishing HMOs. One can imagine the corporate executive requesting an opinion of such an undertaking from legal counsel and receiving a conservative warning that medical malpractice might subject the corporation to millions of dollars in settlement costs beyond the limits of malpractice insurance available to the physician employees. General Electric and DuPont decided against sponsoring HMOs for just this reason. At least as important a problem is the concern some corporations have about their company image should a malpractice case lead to bad publicity.

Another factor that has discouraged some business corporations from entering the HMO movement is a perceived difficulty in recruiting physicians. Doctors appear to be busy in their medical practices and earning significant incomes and seem to have little incentive to become part of the HMOs of business corporations.

All of these concerns, however, appear to be without much foundation. Medical malpractice is a serious problem, but not an insurmountable one; moreover, insulating the parent corporation from the HMO sufficiently to protect the assets of the parent company is possible. Entering the health care industry probably provides a favorable public image that would offset much of the unfavorable publicity that would accompany a medical mishap.

Moreover, conditions are favorable for recruiting physicians into HMOs. In the past ten years, the number of medical schools in the country has increased by 37 percent, from 84 schools in 1965 to 115 at present. The total graduating medical class for 1976 was 13,470 students, an increase of 81 percent over 1965.[13] In addition, 17.5 percent of the nation's newly licensed physicians in 1960 were graduates of foreign medical schools. By 1974, the percentage had risen to 40 percent.[14] A young physician today also faces significant expense and, frequently, years of effort to establish a medical practice. Many specialists are required not only to borrow heavily to finance their medical educations, but to finance the development of their practices as well. In parts of the country medical malpractice insurance for some specialists costs over $30,000 the first year.

Moreover, today bank loans to establish a practice are not always available. Under these circumstances, employment with a corporation may be attractive, at least until the young physician has been able to save some funds and reduce his debts from medical training. Some business corporations view the growing numbers of physicians who find it difficult to penetrate the private practice market as the key to developing medical staffs and beginning a medical business.

Ultimately, of course, the participation of business corporations in HMOs will depend on their assessment of the profitability of managing prepaid health plans. Some corporations have concluded that they can make only 6 to 7 percent return per year on their investment in an HMO and have decided to look elsewhere for business opportunities. Given the inefficiency in American medicine, however, it is unlikely that all business corporations will come to such a pessimistic conclusion. Success in health care will depend on providing quality health care more effectively than has been done in the inefficient fee-for-service sector.

As Congress passes new legislation to make it easier for HMOs to qualify under federal law, the attractiveness of HMOs as business investments will be considerably enhanced.

CONCLUSION

Consider the following comments on the U.S. health care delivery system that appeared in a *Reader's Digest* article:

> The public does not believe that medicine is evolving satisfactorily. It does not blame the medical profession as a whole, but believes that the distribution of medical care is lagging far behind the *science* of medicine. . . . and it is willing to pay more, in total, for medical care if the burden is more fairly distributed, and if the doctors will organize themselves to give more efficient service. . . .
>
> What worries the average man is not the ordinary doctors' bills. The thing that preys on his mind is the unpredictable serious illnesses, with their consultations, specialists, hospitals and surgeons' fees. . . .
>
> The patient has no way of judging for himself the quality of the service he is getting. If the specialist recommends an expensive treatment or operation, the big fee draws a veil of distrust between doctor and patient. The result may be an unnecessary operation; even worse, it may cause a patient to decline an operation which would save his life. . . .
>
> Dr. Richard C. Cabot of Boston has had 40 years' experience in general and hospital practice and as professor of Clinical Medicine at the Harvard Medical School, Dr. Cabot recently said:

> We would never put a judge on the bench under conditions such that he might be influenced by pecuniary considerations. Suppose that if the judge were to hand down one decision he got $5,000, and if he decided the other way he got nothing. But we allow the private practitioner to face this sort of temptation.
>
> The greatest single curse in medicine is the curse of unnecessary operations, and there would be fewer of them if the doctor got the same salary whether he operated or not. . . . I maintain that to have doctors working on salary would be better for doctors as well as for patients.

This language aptly describes problems of the present health care delivery system. Yet it was written in 1938.[15]

Health care planners, politicians, health economists, medical societies, health insurance companies, labor unions, and consumer interest groups debate endlessly about the need to reform health care delivery in the United States. Yet instead of reform we get little more than additional funding pumped into the present delivery system. The student of history may well conclude, therefore, that the future will not be much different from the past.

A reasonable forecast for the future would thus seem to be the following. Fee-for-service health care will continue to dominate American medicine; national health insurance will be enacted, will prove to be expensive and inflationary, and will lead to efforts to cut back eligibility and to control fees; new but ineffectual regulations will be attempted as each of a series of Undersecretaries of Health at the Department of Health, Education, and Welfare attempts to leave his personal mark on American health care delivery. A hopeful solution is that the HMO movement will gain momentum, but that will depend largely on the success of Congress's attempts to amend the 1973 HMO Act to allow HMOs to offer economically viable health plans. Yet, despite all the attention that has been paid to reform of health care delivery over the past four decades, one should not be surprised if penetration of the health care industry by business corporations turned out to be society's most effective instrument for curtailing unnecessary care and containing health care costs.

Notes

CHAPTER 1

1. M. S. Mueller and R. M. Gibson, "National Health Expenditures, Fiscal Year 1975," *Social Security Bulletin*, vol. 39, no. 2 (February 1976), p. 5.

2. Council on Wage and Price Stability, Executive Office of the President, Staff Report, *The Problem of Rising Health Care Costs*, Washington, D.C., April 1976, p. ii.

3. Bureau of Labor Statistics, U.S. Department of Labor, *Handbook of Labor Statistics 1975—Reference Edition*, Washington, D.C., 1975, Table 128; Bureau of Labor Statistics, *The Consumer Price Index*, Washington, D.C., various monthly issues.

4. Council on Wage and Price Stability, *The Problem of Rising Health Care Costs*, p. iii.

CHAPTER 2

1. American Medical Association, *Horizons Unlimited: A Handbook Describing Rewarding Career Opportunities in Medicine and Allied Fields* (Chicago: American Medical Association, 1970), p. 8.

2. V. L. Wilson, editor, *Medical School Admission Requirements, 1975-76, U.S.A. and Canada* (Washington, D.C.: Association of American Medical Colleges, 1974), p. 3.

3. J. Ellard, "The Disease of Being a Doctor," *Medical Journal of Australia*, vol. 2 (August 31, 1974), p. 319.

4. Ibid., p. 319.

5. C. D. Townes, Jr., "The Doctor's Image of Himself," *Minnesota Medicine* (April 1974), p. 315.

6. L. P. Levitt, "The Personality of the Medical Student," *Chicago Medical School Quarterly*, vol. 25, no. 4 (Winter 1966), pp. 204-205.

7. American Medical Association, *Socioeconomic Issues of Health, 1975-76* (Chicago: Center for Health Services Research and Development, American Medical Association, 1976), p. 194.

8. A. E. Crowley, editor, "Medical Education in the United States, 1974-75," *Journal of the American Medical Association*, vol. 234, no. 13 (December 1975), p. 1339.

9. American Medical Association, *Socioeconomic Issues*, pp. 61-62.

10. American Medical Association, *Profile of Medical Practice, 1975-76* (Chicago: Center for Health Services Research and Development, American Medical Association, 1976), p. 93.

11. Ibid., pp. 102-05.

12. American Medical Association, *Socioeconomic Issues*, p. 69.

13. J. Colombotos, "Social Origins and Ideology of Physicians: A Study of the Effects of Early Socialization," *Journal of Health and Social Behavior*, vol. 10 (March 16-29, 1969), p. 17.

14. Crowley, "Medical Education," p. 1345.

15. J. L. Evans, "Psychiatric Illness in the Physician's Wife," *American Journal of Psychiatry*, vol. 122 (August 1965), p. 159.

16. L. I. Dublin and M. Spiegleman, "Longevity and Mortality of Physicians," *Journal of the American Medical Association*, vol. 134, no. 15 (August 9, 1974), p. 1214.

17. D. H. Blankenhorn, C. D. Jenkins, W. Insull, Jr., and L. Weiss, "Type A Physicians and Coronary Risk Education," *Annals of Internal Medicine*, vol. 81, no. 5 (November 1974), pp. 700-01.

18. American Medical Association, *Profile of Medical Practice, 1974* (Chicago: Center for Health Services Research and Development, American Medical Association, 1974), p. 86.

19. J. J. Hanlon, "Suicide," Chapter 24 in *Public Health: Administration and Practice* (Saint Louis: C. V. Mosby Co., 1974), p. 450.

20. A Report of the AMA Council on Mental Health, "The Sick Physician, Impairment by Psychiatric Disorders, Including Alcoholism and Drug Dependence," *Journal of the American Medical Association*, vol. 223, no. 6 (February 5, 1973), p. 685.

21. Ibid., pp. 684-85.

22. W. A. Cramond, "Anxiety in Medical Practice," *Australian Journal of Psychiatry*, vol. 3 (November 1969), p. 324.

23. D. Maddison, "Stress on the Doctor and His Family," *Medical Journal of Australia*, vol. 2 (August 31, 1974), p. 316.

24. G. E. Vaillant, N. Sobowale, and C. McArthur, "Some Psychologic Vulnerabilities of Physicians," *New England Journal of Medicine* (August 24, 1972), pp. 372-75.

25. L. M. Terman, "Scientists and Non-Scientists in a Group of 800 Gifted Men," *Psychological Monographs*, vol. 68, no. 7 (1954), p. 34.

26. M. Rosenberg, *Occupations and Values* (New York: The Free Press of Glencoe, 1957), pp. 10-35.

27. E. Freidson, "The Clinical Mentality," *Profession of Medicine: A Study of the Sociology of Applied Knowledge* (New York: Dodd, Mead, 1970), p. 174.

28. National Opinion Research Center, *Career Preferences of Medical Students in the United States*, Study in Conjunction with Office of the Surgeon General, Dept. of the Army, Publication No. DA 49007MD 719, Chicago, 1956.

29. J. Colombotos, "Social Origins," p. 20.

30. G. D. Otis and J. R. Weiss, "Patterns of Medical Career Preference," *Journal of Medical Education*, vol. 48 (December 1973), p. 116.

31. American Medical Association, *Socioeconomic Issues of Health, 1974* (Chicago: Center for Health Services Research and Development, American Medical Association, 1975), p. 17.

32. Ibid., pp. 36–41; and K. A. Heald, J. K. Cooper, and S. Coleman, *Choice of Location or Practice of Medical School Graduates: Analysis of Two Surveys* (Santa Monica, Calif.: The Rand Corporation, 1974), pp. 26–27.

33. American Medical Association, *Socioeconomic Issues of Health, 1974*, pp. 22–28.

CHAPTER 3

1. American Medical Association, *Profile of Medical Practice, 1975–76* (Chicago: Center for Health Services Research and Development, American Medical Association, 1976), p. 152.

2. "My Doctor, the Corporation," *New York Times Magazine* (December 29, 1974), pp. 8–9.

CHAPTER 4

1. U. E. Reinhardt, *Physician Productivity and the Demand for Health Manpower* (Cambridge, Mass.: Ballinger Publishing Company, 1975), p. 107.

2. Ibid., p. 110.

3. Ibid., p. 111.

4. U. E. Reinhardt, "A Production Function for Physician Services," *Review of Economics and Statistics*, vol. 54, no. 1 (February 1972), p. 64.

5. L. J. Kimbell and R. T. Deane, "Analysis of the Utilization of Ancillary Personnel Using Production Functions," *An Original Comparative Economic Analysis of Group Practice and Solo Fee-For-Service Practice: Final Report; Analyses from the Seventh Periodic Survey of Physicians*, Human Resources Research Center, University of Southern California, January 31, 1974 (available from National Technical Information Service, Springfield, Va., as PB 241 546), pp. 26–45.

6. W. B. Schwartz, Testimony in *Hearings* before the Subcommittee on Health of the Committee on Labor and Public Welfare, U.S. Senate, 92nd Congress, First Session, on Examination of the Health Care Crisis in America, Part 3, Washington, D.C., May 10, 1971, p. 448, as cited in Reinhardt, *Physician Productivity*, pp. 108–109.

7. R. Zeckhauser and M. Eliastam, "The Productivity Potential of the Physician Assistant," *Journal of Human Resources*, vol. 9, no. 1 (Winter 1974), p. 95.

8. D. R. Ostergard, E. M. Broen, and J. R. Marshall, "The Family Planning Specialist as a Provider of Health Care Services," *Fertility and Sterility*, vol. 23, no. 7 (July 1972), p. 506.

9. E. C. Nelson, A. R. Jacobs, and K. G. Johnson, "Patients' Acceptance of Physician Assistants," *Journal of the American Medical Association*, vol. 228, no. 1 (April 1, 1974), pp. 63–67.

10. Reinhardt, "A Production Function for Physician Services," p. 63; Kimbell and Deane, "Analysis of the Utilization of Ancillary Personnel using Production Functions," pp. 26–45.

11. Zeckhauser and Eliastam, "The Productivity Potential of the Physician Assistant," p. 95.

CHAPTER 5

1. W. B. Schwartz, "Medicine and the Computer," *New England Journal of Medicine*, vol. 283 (December 1970), p. 1258, cited in U. E. Reinhardt, *Physician Productivity and the Demand for Health Manpower: An Economic Analysis* (Cambridge, Mass.: Ballinger Publishing Company, 1975), pp. 105–06.

2. Reinhardt, ibid., pp. 106–07.

CHAPTER 6

1. U. E. Reinhardt, *Physician Productivity and the Demand for Health Manpower: An Economic Analysis* (Cambridge, Mass.: Ballinger Publishing Company, 1975), pp. 92–93.

2. Rashi Fein, *The Doctor Shortage: An Economic Diagnosis* (Washington, D.C.: The Brookings Institution, 1967), p. 98.

3. J. Newhouse, "The Economics of Group Practice," *Journal of Human Resources*, vol. 8, no. 1 (Winter 1973), pp. 37–56.

4. R. M. Bailey, "Economies of Scale in Outpatient Medical Practice," *Group Practice* (July 1968), pp. 24–33.

5. R. L. Ernst and H. J. Schwartz, "Determinants of the Costs of Physicians' Services," in *An Original Comparative Economic Analysis of Group Practice and Solo Fee-For-Service Practice: Final Report; Analyses from the Seventh Periodic Survey of Physicians*, Human Resources Research Center, University of Southern California, January 31, 1974 (available from National Technical Information Service, Springfield, Va., as PB 241 546), p. 271.

6. Newhouse, "The Economics of Group Practice."

7. F. L. Golladay, M. E. Manser, and K. R. Smith, "Scale Economies in the Delivery of Medical Care: A Mixed Integer Programming Analysis of Efficient Manpower Utilization," *Journal of Human Resources*, vol. 9, no. 1 (Winter 1974), pp. 50–62.

8. R. L. Ernst and H. J. Schwartz, "Cost Functions for Physicians' Practice: Evidence on Economies of Scale," in *An Original and Comparative Economic Analysis*, pp. 522–636; and "Determinants of the Costs of Physicians' Services," in *An Original and Comparative Economic Analysis*, pp. 255–336.

9. Ernst and Schwartz, "Cost Functions."

10. Ernst and Schwartz, "Determinants of the Costs."

11. Ibid., p. 258.

12. Ibid., p. 319.

13. American Medical Association, *Profile of Medical Practice, 1975-76* (Chicago: Center for Health Services Research and Development, American Medical Association, 1976), p. 11.

14. Ibid., pp. 16-18.

15. National Advisory Commission on Health Manpower, *Report of the Commission*, 2 vols., Washington, D.C., 1967, vol. 2, pp. 215-16.

16. Ernst and Schwartz, "Cost Functions," p. 555.

CHAPTER 7

1. American Medical Association, *Profile of Medical Practice, 1975-76* (Chicago: Center for Health Services Research and Development, American Medical Association, 1976), p. 128.

2. Ibid., p. 168.

3. E. Freidson and B. Rhea, "Processes of Control in a Company of Equals," *Social Problems*, vol. 2, no. 2 (1963), pp. 119-31.

4. American Medical Association, *Socioeconomic Issues of Health, 1975-76*, (Chicago: Center for Health Services Research and Development, American Medical Association, 1976), p. 128.

5. American Medical Association, *Profile of Medical Practice, 1975-76*, p. 13.

6. Ibid., p. 21.

CHAPTER 8

1. C. M. Lindsay, "Real Returns to Medical Education," *Journal of Human Resources*, vol. 8, no. 3 (Summer 1973), pp. 331-48.

2. M. S. Feldstein, "Econometric Studies of Health Economics," in M. D. Intriligator and D. A. Kendrick, *Frontiers of Quantitative Economics*, vol. II (Amsterdam: North-Holland Publishing Company, 1974), pp. 414-415.

3. R. A. Kessel, "Price Discrimination in Medicine, *Journal of Law and Economics*, vol. 1 (October 1958), pp. 20-54.

4. *California Relative Value Studies* (San Francisco: California Medical Association, 1975).

5. *Official Minimum Medical Fee Schedule—Division of Industrial Accidents of the State of California* (San Francisco: Sutter Publications, 1972).

6. *American Medical News* (July 26, 1976), p. 1.

CHAPTER 9

1. K. Davis, *National Health Insurance: Benefits, Costs, and Consequences* (Washington, D.C.: The Brookings Institution, 1975), pp. 14-17.

2. B. M. Mitchell and C. E. Phelps, *Employer-paid Group Health Insurance and the Costs of Mandated National Coverage*, R-1509-HEW (Santa Monica, Calif.: The Rand Corporation, 1975), p. 17.

3. B. S. Cooper, N. L. Worthington, and P. A. Piro, "National Health Expenditures, 1929-1973," *Social Security Bulletin*, vol. 37, no. 2 (February 1974), Table 6, p. 15.

4. Mitchell and Phelps, *Employer-paid Group Health*, p. 2.

5. G. S. Goldstein and M. V. Pauly, "Group Health Insurance as a Local Public Good," in R. N. Rosett, editor, *The Role of Health Insurance in the Health Services Sector*, for National Bureau of Economic Research (New York: Neale Watson Academic Publications, 1976).

6. R. G. Beck, "The Effects of Co-payment on the Poor," *Journal of Human Resources*, vol. 9, no. 1 (Winter 1974), pp. 129-42.

7. M. S. Feldstein, "The Welfare Loss of Excess Health Insurance," *Journal of Political Economy*, vol. 81, no. 2, Part 1 (March-April 1973), p. 252.

8. J. H. Knowles, "Where Doctors Fail," *Saturday Review* (August 22, 1970), p. 21.

9. American Medical Association, *Socioeconomic Issues of Health, 1975-76* (Chicago: Center for Health Services Research and Development, American Medical Association, 1976), p. 155.

10. B. H. Kehrer, "The Physician as Purchasing Agent for His Patient," in American Medical Association, B. S. Eisenberg and P. Aherne, eds., *Socioeconomic Issues of Health Care, 1974* (Chicago: Center for Health Services Research and Development, American Medical Association, 1974), pp. 55-61. Reprinted by permission of the American Medical Association.

11. V. R. Fuchs, "The Growing Demand for Medical Care," in V. R. Fuchs, ed., *Essays in the Economics of Health and Medical Care* (New York: Columbia University Press, 1972), p. 66.

12. W. G. Smith, "The Malpractice Crisis and the Insurance Carrier," *Transactions of the American Academy of Ophthalmology and Otolaryngology*, vol. 80, no. 3 (May-June 1975), p. 286.

13. H. S. Denenberg, "The Medical Malpractice Mess," *The Progressive* (May 1975), p. 20.

14. C. W. Weinberger, "Malpractice—A National View," *Arizona Medicine*, vol. 32, no. 2 (February 1975), p. 117.

15. See Notes 19 through 27.

16. M. Silverman and P. R. Lee, *Pills, Profits and Politics* (Berkeley: University of California Press, 1974), p. 167.

17. Ibid., p. 54.

18. T. D. Rucker, "Economic Problems in Drug Distribution," *Inquiry*, vol. 9, no. 3 (September 1972), p. 43.

19. E. G. McCarthy and G. W. Widner, "Effect of Screening by Consultants on Recommended Elective Surgical Procedures," *New England Journal of Medicine*, vol. 291 (December 19, 1974), p. 1331.

20. S. M. Wolfe, Testimony in *Hearings* before the Subcommittee on Oversight and Investigations on Unnecessary Surgery of the Interstate and Foreign Commerce Committee, House of Representatives, 94th Congress, 1st Session, Washington, D.C., July 15, 1975 (mimeo), p. 6.

21. J. P. Bunker, "A Comparison of Operations and Surgeons in the United

States and in England and Wales," *New England Journal of Medicine*, vol. 282 (January 15, 1970), p. 135.

22. C. F. Gaus, B. S. Cooper, and C. G. Hirschman, "Contrasts in HMO and Fee-for-Service Performance," *Social Security Bulletin*, vol. 39, no. 5 (May 1976), pp. 3-14.

23. J. C. Doyle, "Unnecessary Hysterectomies," *Journal of the American Medical Association*, vol. 151, no. 5 (January 31, 1954), p. 360.

24. Wolfe, Testimony, p. 2.

CHAPTER 10

1. E. M. Burns, "The Role of Government in Health Services," *Bulletin of the New York Academy of Medicine*, vol. 41, no. 7 (July 1965), p. 786.

2. Ibid., p. 792.

3. W. A. Glaser, *Paying the Doctor* (Baltimore, Md.: The Johns Hopkins Press, 1970), pp. 136-37.

4. K. Davis, *National Health Insurance* (Washington, D.C.: The Brookings Institution, 1975), Chapter 5.

5. Editorial, *The New York Times* (August 17, 1969).

6. J. P. Newhouse, C. E. Phelps, and W. B. Schwartz, "Policy Options and the Impact of National Health Insurance," *New England Journal of Medicine*, vol. 290, no. 24 (June 13, 1974), p. 1358.

7. W. M. McClure, cited in A. C. Enthoven, "Can We Control the Cost of Health Care?" *The Stanford Magazine*, vol. 3, no. 2 (November 1975), p. 14.

8. D. Neuhauser and W. Halperin, *Cost-Effective Clinical Decision Making*, Cases in Health Series No. 3B (Boston: Harvard School of Public Health and Center for Community Health and Medical Care, 1973).

9. J. Enoch Powell, *Medicine and Politics* (London: Pitman Medical Publishing Co., 1966), Chapter 4.

10. Department of Health, Education and Welfare, *Forward Plan for Health FY 1977-81*, Washington, D.C., June, 1975, p. 163.

11. M. Obledo, from a letter to Casper W. Weinberger, Secretary of the Department of Health, Education and Welfare, July 9, 1975, p. 3.

12. Cambridge Research Institute, *Trends Affecting the U.S. Health Care System* (Cambridge, Mass.: Cambridge Research Institute, 1975), pp. 11-36.

13. H. S. Denenberg, "The Medical Malpractice Mess," *The Progressive* (May 1975), p. 20.

14. G. Pickett, from a presentation at the conference "Toward a National Health Policy," sponsored by the National Association of Regional Medical Programs, Atlanta, May 6, 1975.

15. C. R. Gaus, B. S. Cooper, and C. G. Hirschman, "Contrasts in HMO and Fee-for-Service Performance," *Social Security Bulletin*, vol. 39, no. 5 (May 1976).

16. L. J. Warshaw, "The HMO Concept and Its Current Status," *Journal of Occupational Medicine*, vol. 17, no. 10 (October 1975), p. 630.

17. S. R. Garfield, "A New Medical Care Delivery System Model," *Proceed-*

ings of an International Conference on Health Technology Systems (Potomac, Md.: Operations Research Society of America, 1974), p. 130.

18. P. Starr, "The Undelivered Health System," *The Public Interest* (Winter 1976), pp. 78-79.

19. Ibid., p. 79.

CHAPTER 11

1. C. C. Havighurst, "Health Maintenance Organization and the Market for Health Services," *Law and Contemporary Problems*, vol. 35 (Autumn 1970), p. 740.

2. Ibid., pp. 739-40.

3. R. Stevens, *American Medicine and the Public Interest* (New Haven, Conn.: Yale University Press, 1971), p. 422.

4. M. Friedman, *Capitalism and Freedom* (Chicago: University of Chicago Press, 1963), p. 154.

5. S. S. Goldwater, "Medical Practice and Hospitalization," *Hospitals* (July 1938), pp. 11-12.

6. A. W. Willcox, "Hospitals and the Corporate Practice of Medicine," *Cornell Law Quarterly*, vol. 45 (1960), pp. 436, 486.

7. Ibid., p. 449.

8. Ibid., pp. 456-57.

9. *Complete Service Bureau v. San Diego County Medical Society*, 43 Ca. 2d 201, 208 (1954), cited in the Opinion of Evelle J. Younger, Attorney General, State of California, No. CV 71/207 (March 3, 1972).

10. Musick, Peeler & Garrett, Attorneys for the California Hospital Association, from a letter addressed to Evelle J. Younger, Attorney General, State of California, dated April 14, 1972, p. 1.

11. The Conference Board, *Industry Roles in Health Care* (New York: The Conference Board, 1974), p. 64.

12. Willcox, "Hospitals and the Corporate Practice," p. 402

13. A. E. Crowley, "Medical Education in the United States 1974-75," *Journal of the American Medical Association*, vol. 234, no. 13 (December 1975), p. 1338. Data for 1975-76 are preliminary estimates of the Association of American Medical Colleges.

14. American Medical Association, *Socioeconomic Issues of Health, 1975-76* (Chicago: Center for Health Services Research and Development, American Medical Association, 1976), pp. 200-01.

15. B. Smith, "Diagnosing the Doctors," *The Reader's Digest*, vol. 33, no. 196 (August 1938), pp. 1-5.

Bibliography

Abel-Smith, Brian. "Value for Money in Health Services." *Social Security Bulletin*, vol. 37 (July 1974), pp. 17–28.

a'Brook, M. F., J. D. Hailstone, and I. E. J. McLauchlan. "Psychiatric Illness in the Medical Profession." *British Journal of Psychiatry*, vol. 113 (1967), pp. 1013-23.

Alexander, C. A. "The Effects of Change in Method of Paying Physicians: The Baltimore Experience." *American Journal of Public Health*, vol. 57, no. 8 (August 1967), pp. 1278-89.

American Hospital Association. *Governance of Health Care Institutions*. Catalog No. G001.10M-11/74-4103, 2M-7175-4589. Chicago: American Hospital Association, 1974.

——. *Guidelines for Resolution of Conflicts of Interest in Health Care Institutions*. Chicago: American Hospital Association, 1974.

American Medical Association. A Report of the AMA Council on Mental Health, "The Sick Physician, Impairment by Psychiatric Disorders, Including Alcoholism and Drug Dependence." *Journal of the American Medical Association*, vol. 223, no. 6 (February 5, 1973), pp. 684-87.

——. *Horizons Unlimited: A Handbook Describing Rewarding Career Opportunities in Medicine and Allied Fields*. Chicago: American Medical Association, 1970.

——. *Profile of Medical Practice, 1974*, Judith Warner and Phil Aherne, eds. Chicago: Center for Health Services Research and Development, American Medical Association, 1975.

——. *Profile of Medical Practice, 1975-76*, James R. Cantwell, ed. Chicago: Center for Health Services Research and Development, American Medical Association, 1976.

——. *Socioeconomic Issues of Health, 1974*, Barry S. Eisenberg and Phil

Aherne, eds. Chicago: Center for Health Services Research and Development, American Medical Association, 1975.

———. *Socioeconomic Issues of Health, 1975–76,* Henry R. Mason, ed. Chicago: Center for Health Services Research and Development, American Medical Association, 1976.

Anderson, Odin W. *Health Care: Can There Be Equity? The United States, Sweden, and England.* New York: John Wiley & Sons, 1972.

Anderson, Ronald, Richard Foster, and Peter Weil. "Rates and Correlates of Expenditure Increases for Personal Health Services: Pre- and Post-Medicare and Medicaid." *Inquiry,* vol. 13, no. 2 (June 1976), pp. 136–44.

Andreano, Ralph L., and Burton A. Weisbrod. *American Health Policy.* Chicago: Rand McNally College Publishing Company, 1974.

Angermeier, Ingo. "Impact of Community Rating and Open Enrollment on a Prepaid Group Practice." *Inquiry* vol. 13, no. 1 (March 1976), pp. 48–53.

"A Private Manager for Medicaid." *Business Week* (May 19, 1975), pp. 45–46.

Arrow, Kenneth J. "Uncertainty and the Welfare Economics of Medical Care." *American Economic Review,* vol. 53 (December 1963), pp. 941–73.

Association of American Medical Colleges. *Undergraduate Medical Education, Elements—Objectives—Costs, Report of the Commission on the Financing of Medical Education.* Washington, D.C.: Association of American Medical Colleges, 1973.

Avorn, Jerry. "The Future of Doctoring." *The New York Times Magazine* (December 29, 1974), pp. 71–79.

"A Way to Clean up the Malpractice Mess." *Business Week* (February 24, 1975), pp. 30–32.

Bailey, Richard M. "An Economist's View of the Health Services Industry." *Inquiry,* vol. 6, no. 1 (March 1969), pp. 3–18.

———. "Appraisal of Experience in Fee-for-Service Group Practice in the San Francisco Bay Area: A Comparison of Internists in Solo and Group Practice." Presented to the Health Conference of the New York Academy of Medicine, April 1968.

———. "Economies of Scale in Medical Practice." In Herbert E. Klarman, ed., *Empirical Studies in Health Economics,* Proceedings of the Second Conference on the Economics of Health. Baltimore, Md.: The Johns Hopkins Press, 1970.

———. "Economies of Scale in Outpatient Medical Practice." *Group Practice* (July 1968), pp. 24–33.

Bailey, Richard M., and Thomas M. Tierney, Jr. "Costs, Service Differences, and Prices in Private Clinical Laboratories." *The Milbank Memorial Fund Quarterly,* vol. 52 (Summer 1974), pp. 265–89.

Baird, C. W. "A Proposal for Financing the Purchase of Health Services." *Journal of Human Resources,* vol. 9, no. 4 (Winter 1970), pp. 89–105.

Ballenger, Martha D. "Physician's Assistants and the Licensing Issue." *Monthly Labor Review,* vol. 94, no. 4 (April 1971), pp. 62–63.

Baron, David P. "A Study of Hospital Cost Inflation." *Journal of Human Resources,* vol. 9, no. 1 (Winter 1974), pp. 33–49.

Beck, R. G. "The Effects of Co-Payment on the Poor." *Journal of Human Resources*, vol. 9, no. 1 (Winter 1974), pp. 129-42.

Benham, L., A. Maurizi, and M. W. Reder. "Location and Migration of Medics: Physicians and Dentists." *Review of Economics and Statistics*, vol. 50, no. 3 (August 1968), pp. 332-47.

Berki, Sylvester E. *Hospital Economics: Studies in Social and Economic Process.* Lexington, Mass.: D. C. Heath, 1972.

Berry, Ralph E., Jr. "Cost and Efficiency in the Production of Hospital Services." *Milbank Memorial Fund Quarterly*, vol. 52 (Summer 1974), pp. 291-313.

——. "Perspectives on Rate Regulation." Presented at the Conference on Regulation in the Health Industry sponsored by the Institute of Medicine, National Academy of Sciences, Washington, D.C., January 7-9, 1974.

Blachly, P. H., William Disher, and Gregory Roduner. "Suicide by Physicians." *Bulletin of Suicidology*, December 1968.

Blair, Roger D., Jerry R. Jackson, and Ronald J. Vogel. "Economies of Scale in the Administration of Health Insurance." *Review of Economics and Statistics*, vol. 57, no. 2 (May 1975), pp. 185-89.

Blankenhorn, David H., C. David Jenkins, William Insull, Jr., and Leona Weiss. "Type-A Physicians and Coronary Risk Education." *Annals of Internal Medicine*, vol. 81 (November 1974), pp. 700-01.

Bloom, Samuel W. "The Process of Becoming a Physician." *Annals of the American Academy of Political and Social Science*, vol. 346 (1963).

Blumberg, Mark S. *Trends and Projections of Physicians in the United States, 1967-2002.* A Technical Report Sponsored by the Carnegie Commission on Higher Education. Berkeley, Calif.: The Carnegie Foundation for the Advancement of Teaching, 1971.

Boan, J. A. *Group Practice.* Study prepared for the Royal Commission on Health Services, 1964. Ottawa: Queen's Printer, 1966.

Boness, Fredrick. "Legal Constraints on the Utilization of Allied Health Personnel," Discussion Paper 73-6. La Jolla, Calif.: Institute of Policy Analysis, October 1973.

Brewster, Agnes W., and Estelle Seldowitz. "Medical Society Relative Value Scales and the Medical Market." *Public Health Reports*, vol. 80 (June 1965), pp. 501-10.

Brown, Douglas, Martin Feldstein, and Harvey Lapan. "The Rising Price of Physicians' Services: A Clarification." *Review of Economics and Statistics*, vol. 56 (August 1974), pp. 396-98.

Brown, Douglas M., and Harvey E. Lapan. "The Rising Price of Physicians' Services: A Comment." *Review of Economic Statistics*, vol. 54 (February 1972), pp. 101-05.

Buck M. L. *How to Build a More Rewarding Medical Practice.* Englewood Cliffs, N. J.: Executive Reports Corporation, 1974.

Bunker, John P. "A Comparison of Operations and Surgeons in the United States and in England and Wales." *New England Journal of Medicine*, vol. 282 (January 15, 1970), pp. 135-44.

Bureau of Labor Statistics, U.S. Department of Labor. *Handbook of Labor Statistics, 1975—Reference Edition.* Washington, D.C.: U.S. Government Printing Office, 1975.

——. *The Consumer Price Index.* Washington, D.C.: U.S. Government Printing Office, various monthly issues.

Burns, Eveline M. *Health Services for Tomorrow: Trends and Issues.* New York: Dunellen, 1973.

Butter, Irene. "Health Manpower Research: A Survey." *Inquiry,* vol. 4 (December 1967), pp. 5–41.

Butter, Irene, and Richard Schaffner. "Foreign Medical Graduates and Equal Access to Medical Care." *Medical Care,* vol. 9 (1971), pp. 136–43.

California Medical Association. *California Relative Value Studies.* San Francisco: California Medical Association, 1975.

Cambridge Research Institute. *Trends Affecting the U.S. Health Care System.* Cambridge, Mass.: Cambridge Research Institute, 1975.

Carnegie Commission on Higher Education. *Higher Education and the Nation's Health: Policies for Medical and Dental Education.* New York: McGraw-Hill Book Co., 1970.

Carnegie Council on Policy Studies. *Progress and Problems in Medical and Dental Education.* San Francisco: Jossey-Bass Publishers, 1976.

Chapman, C. B., and J. M. Talmadge. "Historical and Political Background of Federal Health Care Legislation." *Law and Contemporary Problems,* vol. 35, no. 2 (Spring 1970), pp. 334–47.

Cochrane, Archibald L. *Efficiency and Effectiveness.* London: Nuffield Provincial Hospitals Trust, 1972.

Coe, Rodney M., and Leonard Fichtenbaum. "Utilization of Physician Assistants: Some Implications for Medical Practice." *Medical Care,* vol. 10 (November-December 1972), pp. 497–504.

Cohen, Harris C. "Professional Licensure, Organizational Behavior, and the Public Interest." *Milbank Memorial Fund Quarterly, Health and Society,* vol. 51, no. 1 (Winter 1973), pp. 73–88.

Colombotos, John. "Social Origins and Ideology of Physicians: A Study of the Effects of Early Socialization." *Journal of Health and Social Behavior,* vol. 10 (March 1969), pp. 16–29.

Commission on the Cost of Medical Care. *General Report.* Chicago: American Medical Association, 1964.

Committee for Economic Development, Research and Policy Committee. *Building a National Health-Care System.* New York: Committee for Economic Development, 1973.

Condit, G. W. *Syllabus for Office Practice.* New York: Economedic Publishing Corporation, 1967.

Cooper, Barbara S., and Paula A Piro. "Age Differences in Medical Care Spending, Fiscal Year 1973." *Social Security Bulletin,* vol. 37 (May 1974), pp. 3–14, 29–31, 40.

Cooper, Barbara S., and Dorothy P. Rice. "The Economic Cost of Illness Revisited." *Social Security Bulletin,* vol. 39, no. 2 (February 1976), pp. 21–36.

Cooper, Barbara S., and Nancy L. Worthington. "National Health Expenditures, 1929–72." *Social Security Bulletin,* vol. 36, no. 1 (January 1973), pp. 3–19.

Cooper, Barbara S., Nancy L. Worthington, and P. A. Piro. "National Health

Expenditures, 1929-73." *Social Security Bulletin,* vol. 37, no. 2 (February 1974), pp. 3-19.

Cooper, James K., Karen Heald, Michael Samuels, and Sinclair Coleman. "Rural or Urban Practice: Factors Influencing the Location Decisions of Primary Care Physicians." *Inquiry,* vol. 12, no. 1 (March 1975), pp. 18-25.

Corbin, Mildred, and Aaron Krute. "Some Aspects of Medicare Experience with Group-Practice Prepayment Plans." *Social Security Bulletin,* vol. 38 (March 1975), pp. 3-11.

Corey, Lawrence, Steven E. Saltman, and Michael F. Epstein, eds. *Medicine in a Changing Society.* Saint Louis: The C. V. Mosby Company, 1972.

Cotton, Horace. *Medical Practice Management.* Oradell, N. J.: Medical Economics Book Division, Inc., 1967.

Council on Wage and Price Stability, Executive Office of the President. Staff Report, *The Problem of Rising Health Care Costs.* Washington, D.C., April 1976.

Cramond, W. A. "Anxiety in Medical Practice—The Doctor's Own Anxiety." *Australian and New Zealand Journal of Psychiatry,* vol. 3 (November 1969), pp. 324-29.

Crowley, A. E., ed. "Medical Education in the United States 1974-1975." *Journal of the American Medical Association,* vol. 234, no. 13 (December 1975).

Culyer, A. J. "On the Relative Efficiency of the National Health Service." *Kyklos,* vol. 25, no. 2 (1972), pp. 266-87.

Davis, Karen. "A Theory of Economic Behavior in Non-Profit, Private Hospitals." Unpublished Ph.D. Dissertation, Rice University, Houston, Texas, 1969.

———. "Hospital Costs and the Medicare Program." *Social Security Bulletin,* vol. 36, no. 8 (August 1973), pp. 18-36.

———. "Medicaid Payments and Utilization of Medical Services by the Poor." *Inquiry,* vol. 13, no. 2 (June 1976), pp. 122-35.

———. *National Health Insurance: Benefits, Costs, and Consequences.* Washington, D.C.: The Brookings Institution, 1975.

———. "Relationship of Hospital Prices to Costs." *Applied Economics,* vol. 4 (1971), pp. 115-25.

———. "Theories of Hospital Inflation: Some Empirical Evidence." *Journal of Human Resources,* vol. 8, no. 2 (Spring 1973), pp. 181-201.

Davis, Karen, and Louise B. Russell. "The Substitution of Hospital Outpatient Care for Inpatient Care." *Review of Economics and Statistics,* vol. 54, no. 2 (May 1972), pp. 242-49.

Deane, Robert T., and John B. McFarland. "The Direct Estimation of Demand for Ancillary Personnel in Physicians' Practice." In University of Southern California, Human Resources Research Center, *An Original Comparative Economic Analysis of Group Practice and Solo Fee-for-Service Practice: Final Report.* Prepared for National Center for Health Services Research. Springfield, Va., January 31, 1974.

Denenberg, Herbert S. "The Medical Malpractice Mess." *The Progressive* (May 1975), pp. 19-21.

Densen, Paul M., E. W. Jones, E. Balamuth, and Sam Shapiro, "Prepaid Medical Care and Hospital Utilization in a Dual Choice Situation." *American Journal of Public Health,* vol. 50 (November 1960), pp. 1710-26.

Densen, Paul M., Sam Shapiro, E. W. Jones, and I. Baldinger. "Prepaid Medical Care and Hospital Utilization: Comparison of a Group Practice and a Self-Insurance Situation." *Hospitals*, vol. 36 (November 16, 1962), pp. 62-68, 138.

Department of Health, Education and Welfare. *Forward Plan for Health FY 1977-81*. Washington, D.C.: U.S. Government Printing Office, 1975.

Division of Industrial Accidents of the State of California. *Official Minimum Medical Fee Schedule—Division of Industrial Accidents of the State of California*. San Francisco: Sutter Publications, 1972.

Donabedian, Avedis. "An Evaluation of Prepaid Group Practice." *Inquiry*, vol. 6 (September 1969), pp. 3-27.

———. "Evaluating the Quality of Medical Care." *Milbank Memorial Fund Quarterly*, vol. 64 (July 1966), pp. 166-206.

Dorsey, Joseph L. "The Health Maintenance Organization Act of 1973 (P.L. 93-222) and Prepaid Group Practice Plans." *Medical Care*, vol. 13, no. 1 (January 1975), pp. 1-9.

Douglas-Wilson, I., and Gordon McLachlan, eds. *Health Service Prospects: An International Survey*. London: The Lancet Ltd. and the Nuffield Provincial Hospitals Trust, 1973.

Doyle, Joseph C. "Unnecessary Hysterectomies." *Journal of the American Medical Association*, vol. 151, no. 5 (January 31, 1953), pp. 360-65.

Dube, W. F., and Davis G. Johnson. "Study of U.S. Medical School Applicants, 1972-73." *Journal of Medical Education*, vol. 49 (September 1974), pp. 849-69.

Dublin, Louis I., Mortimer Spiegelman, and Roscoe G. Leland. "Longevity and Mortality of Physicians." *Journal of the American Medical Association*, vol. 134 (August 9, 1947), pp. 1211-15.

Duff, Raymond S., and August B. Hollingshead. *Sickness and Society*. New York: Harper & Row, 1968.

Duffy, John C., and Edward M. Litin. "Psychiatric Morbidity of Physicians." *Journal of the American Medical Association*, vol. 189, no. 13 (September 28, 1964), pp. 97-100.

Easton, Allan. *The Design of a Health Maintenance Organization: A Handbook for Practitioners*. New York: Praeger Publishers, 1975.

Egan, Douglas M. *Physician Productivity, Personnel Utilization, and Physician Income*. Denver: Medical Group Management Association, 1969.

Egan, Richard L. "The AMA, Accreditation, and the Number of Physicians." *Journal of the American Medical Association*, vol. 230, no. 12 (December 23-30, 1974), pp. 1681-82.

Ellard, John. "The Disease of Being a Doctor." *Medical Journal of Australia*, vol. 2, no. 9 (August 1974), pp. 318-23.

Ellwood, Paul M., Jr. "Restructuring the Health Delivery System—Will the Health Maintenance Strategy Work?" In *Health Maintenance Organizations: A Reconfiguration of the Health Services System*. Proceedings of the Thirteenth Annual Symposium on Hospital Affairs, Center for Health Administration Studies, University of Chicago, May 1971, pp. 2-11.

Ellwood, Paul M., Jr., Patrick O'Donoghue, Earl J. Hoagberg, Robert Schneider,

Walter McLure, and Rick J. Carlson. *Comparative Analysis of a Competitive HMO System with Other Health Care Delivery Systems* (mimeographed). Minneapolis: Interstudy, 1971.

Enthoven, Alain C. "Can We Control the Cost of Health Care?" *The Stanford Magazine*, vol. 3, no. 2 (November 1975), pp. 14-19.

Epstein, Steven B. "HMOs and the Law." *Group Practice* (August 1973), pp. 9-15.

Ernst, Richard. "An Note on 'The Economics of Group Practice.'" In University of Southern California, Human Resources Research Center, *An Original Comparative Economic Analysis of Group Practice and Solo Fee-for-Service Practice: Final Report.* Prepared for National Center for Health Services Research, Springfield, Va., January 31, 1974.

Ernst, Richard L. and Herbert J. Schwartz. "Cost Functions for Physicians' Practices: Evidence on Economies of Scale." In University of Southern California, Human Resources Research Center, *An Original Comparative Economic Analysis of Group Practice and Solo Fee-for-Service Practice: Final Report.* Prepared for National Center for Health Services Research, Springfield, Va., January 31, 1974.

———. "Determinants of the Costs of Physicians' Services." In University of Southern California, Human Resources Research Center, *An Original Comparative Economic Analysis of Group Practice and Solo Fee-for-Service Practice: Final Report.* Prepared for National Center for Health Services Research, Springfield, Va., January 31, 1974.

Evans, James L. "Psychiatric Illness in the Physician's Wife." *American Journal of Psychiatry*, vol. 122 (1965), pp. 159-63.

Evans, Robert G. " 'Behavioral' Cost Function for Hospitals." *Canadian Journal of Economics*, vol. 4, no. 2 (May 1971), pp. 198-215.

———. *Price Formation in the Market for Physician's Services in Canada, 1957-1969.* Study prepared for the Prices and Incomes Commission, Canada, 1972. Ottawa: Information Canada, 1973.

Evans, Robert G., E. M. A. Parish, and Floyd Sully. "Medical Productivity, Scale Effects, and Demand Generation." *Canadian Journal of Economics*, vol. 6 (August 1973), pp. 376-93.

Falk, I. S. "Prospects for Prepaid Group Practice." *American Journal of Public Health*, vol. 59 (January 1969).

Fein, Rashi. *The Doctor Shortage: An Economic Diagnosis.* Washington, D.C.: The Brookings Institution, 1967.

Feldman, Marie. "Pediatric Nurse Practitioner's Role in a Large Group Practice." *Hospital Topics*, vol. 50 (March 1972).

Feldstein, Martin S. "An Econometric Model of the Medicare System: Reply." *Quarterly Journal of Economics*, vol. 87, no. 3 (August 1973), pp. 490-94.

———. "Econometric Studies of Health Economics." In M. D. Intrilligator and D. A. Kendrick, eds., *Frontiers of Quantitative Economics.* Amsterdam: North-Holland Publishing Company, 1974, pp. 377-447.

———. *Economic Analysis for Health Service Efficiency: Econometric Studies of the British National Health Service.* Amsterdam: North Holland Publishing Co., 1967.

——. "The Medical Economy." *Scientific American* (September 1973), pp. 151-59.

——. *The Rising Cost of Hospital Care.* Washington, D.C.: Information Resources Press, 1971.

——. "The Rising Price of Physicians' Services." *Review of Economics and Statistics,* vol. 52, no. 2 (May 1970), pp. 121-33.

——. "The Rising Price of Physicians' Services: A Reply." *Review of Economic Statistics,* vol. 54, no. 1 (February 1972), pp. 105-07.

——. "The Welfare Loss of Excess Health Insurance." *Journal of Political Economy,* vol. 81, no. 2, Part 1 (March-April 1973), pp. 251-80.

Feldstein, Paul J. "Research on the Demand for Health Services." *Milbank Memorial Fund Quarterly,* vol. 54 (July 1966, pp. 128-65.

Feldstein, Paul J., and R. M. Severson. "The Demand for Medical Care." In American Medical Association, *Report of the Commission on the Cost of Medical Care,* vol. 1. Chicago: American Medical Association, 1964, pp. 57-76.

Foundation on Employee Health, Medical Care and Welfare. *Family Medical Care under Three Types of Health Insurance* New York: The Foundation on Employee Health, Medical Care and Welfare, 1962.

Frech, H. E. "Ted", III. "The Regulation of Health Insurance and the Medical Market: A Theoretical and Empirical Study," Working Paper in Economics No. 37. Santa Barbara: University of California, Department of Economics, August 1975.

Frech, H. E. "Ted", III, and Paul B. Ginsburg. "Imposed Health Insurance in Monopolistic Markets: A Theoretical Analysis." *Economic Inquiry,* vol. 11 (March 1975), pp. 55-70.

——. "Optimal Scale in Medical Practice: A Survivor Analysis." *The Journal of Business,* vol. 47, no. 1 (January 1974), pp. 23-36.

——. "Physician Pricing: Monopolistic or Competitive: Comment." *Southern Economic Journal,* vol. 38 (April 1972), pp. 573-80.

Freeman, Howard E., Sol Levine, and Leo G. Reeder, eds. *Handbook of Medical Sociology,* 2nd ed. Englewood Cliffs, N. J.: Prentice-Hall, 1972.

Freidson, Eliot. *Profession of Medicine: A Study of the Sociology of Applied Knowledge.* New York: Dodd, Mead, 1973.

Freidson, Eliot, and Judith Lorber, eds. *Medical Men and Their Work.* Chicago: Aldine-Atherton, 1972.

Freidson, Eliot, and Buford Rhea. "Processes of Control in a Company of Equals." In Eliot Freidson and Judith Lorber, eds., *Medical Men and Their Work.* Chicago: Aldine-Atherton, 1972, pp. 185-99.

Friedman, Bernard. "Risk Aversion and the Consumer Choice of Health Insurance Option." *Review of Economics and Statistics,* vol. 56, no. 2 (May 1974), pp. 209-14.

Friedman, Milton. *Capitalism and Freedom.* Chicago: The University of Chicago Press, 1962.

Fuchs, Victor R. "An Economist Looks at Health Care." *Hospital Forum* (March 1976), pp. 6-9.

——, ed. *Essays in the Economics of Health and Medical Care.* Prepared for

National Bureau of Economic Research. New York: Columbia University Press, 1972.

———. "Health Care and the United States Economic System." *Milbank Memorial Fund Quarterly*, vol. 50, no. 2, Part 1 (April 1972), pp. 211–37.

———, ed. *Production and Productivity in the Service Industries.* Prepared for National Bureau of Economic Research, Studies in Income and Wealth, Vol. 34. New York: Columbia University Press, 1969.

———. "The Contribution of Health Services to the American Economy." *Milbank Memorial Fund Quarterly*, vol. 44, no. 4, Part 2 (October 1966), pp. 65–103.

———. "The Growing Demand for Medical Care." *Essays in the Economics of Health and Medical Care.* New York: Columbia University Press, 1972.

———. *Who Shall Live? Health, Economics, and Social Change.* New York: Basic Books, 1974.

Fuchs, Victor R., and Marcia J. Kramer. *Determinants of Expenditures for Physicians' Services in the United States, 1948–68.* Washington, D.C.: National Center for Health Services Research and Development, 1972.

Garfield, Sidney R. "A New Medical Care Delivery System Model." *Proceedings of an International Conference on Health Technology Systems.* Potomac, Md.: Operations Research Society of America, 1974.

———. "The Delivery of Medical Care." *Scientific American*, vol. 222 (April 1970), pp. 15–23.

Garfinkel, Irwin. "Financing Medical Care." *Journal of Human Resources*, vol. 7, no. 2 (Spring 1972), pp. 242–49.

Gaus, Clifton R., Barbara S. Cooper, and Constance G. Hirschman. "Contrasts in HMO and Fee-for-Service Performance." Prepared for Office of Research and Statistics, Social Security Administration. Presented at the American Economic Association Meetings, Dallas, December 30, 1975.

Geist, Robert W. "Incentive Bonuses in Prepayment Plans." *New England Journal of Medicine*, vol. 291, no. 24 (December 12, 1974), pp. 1306–08.

Gerber, Alex. "Author's Reply." *Prism*, vol. 1 (November 1973), pp. 6–7.

———. "The Medical Manpower Shortage." *Journal of Medical Education*, vol. 42 (April 1967), pp. 306–19.

———. "Yes, There Is a Doctor Shortage." *Prism*, vol. 1 (August 1973), pp. 13–15, 60.

Ginsburg, Paul B., and Larry M. Manheim. "Insurance, Copayment, and Health Services Utilization: A Critical Review." *Journal of Economics and Business*, vol. 25 (Spring-Summer 1973), pp. 142–53.

Ginzberg, Eli. "Physician Shortage Reconsidered." *New England Journal of Medicine*, vol. 275 (July 1966), pp. 85–87.

Ginzberg, Eli, and Miriam Ostow. *Men, Money, and Medicine.* New York: Columbia University Press, 1969.

Glaser, William A. *Paying the Doctor: Systems of Remuneration and Their Effects.* Baltimore, Md.: The Johns Hopkins Press, 1970.

Glasgow, John M. "Prepaid Group Practice as a National Health Policy: Problems and Perspectives." *Inquiry*, vol. 9, no. 1 (March 1972), pp. 3–15.

Goldberg, Victor P. "Some Emerging Problems of Prepaid Health Plans in the Medi-Cal System." *Policy Analysis* (Winter 1975), pp. 55–68.

Goldman, Lee. "Factors Related to Physicians' Medical and Political Attitudes: A Documentation of Intraprofessional Variations." *Journal of Health and Social Behavior*, vol. 15, no. 3 (September 1974), pp. 177–87.

Goldstein, Marcus S. *Income of Physicians, Osteopaths, and Dentists from Professional Practice 1965–69*, U.S. Department of Health, Education and Welfare, Social Security Administration, Office of Research and Statistics, DHEW Publication No. (SSA) 73–11852, Staff Paper No. 12. Washington, D.C.: U.S. Government Printing Office, 1972.

Goldwater, S. S. "Medical Practice and Hospitalization." *Hospitals*, vol. 12 (July 1938), pp. 11–16.

Golladay, Fredrick L., Marilyn E. Manser, and Kenneth R. Smith. "Scale Economies in the Delivery of Medical Care: A Mixed Integer Programming Analysis of Efficient Manpower Utilization." *Journal of Human Resources*, vol. 90 (Winter 1974), pp. 50–62.

Gorham, William B. *Medical Care Prices.* Report by the Department of Health, Education and Welfare to the President. Washington, D.C.: U.S. Government Printing Office, February 1967.

Graham, Fred E., III. "Group versus Solo Practice: Arguments and Evidence." *Inquiry*, vol. 9, no. 2 (June 1972), pp. 49–60.

Greenlick, M. R. "The Impact of Prepaid Group Practice on American Medical Care: A Critical Evaluation." *Annals of the American Academy of Political and Social Science.* vol. 399 (January 1972), pp. 100–13.

Gregg, Alan, *For Future Doctors.* Chicago: The University of Chicago Press, 1957.

Gross, Martin L. *The Doctors.* New York: Random House, 1966.

Grossman, Michael. "On the Concept of Health Capital and the Demand for Health." *Journal of Political Economy*, vol. 80, no. 2 (March–April 1972), pp. 223–55.

———. *The Demand for Health: A Theoretical and Empirical Investigation.* New York: Columbia University Press, 1972.

Hanlon, John J. Chapter 6, "Suicide." In *Public Health: Administration and Practice*, 6th Ed. Saint Louis: the C. V. Mosby Co., 1974.

Hansen, W. Lee. "An Appraisal of Physician Manpower Projections." *Inquiry*, vol. 7 (March 1970), pp. 102–13.

Harmer, Ruth M. *American Medical Avarice.* New York: Abelard-Schuman, 1975.

Harris, Richard. *A Sacred Trust.* New York: The New American Library, Inc., 1966.

Harris, Seymour E. *The Economics of American Medicine.* New York: The Macmillan Co., 1964.

———. *The Economics of Health Care.* Berkeley: McCutchan Publishers, 1975.

Harvey, Ernest C., and Leland H. Towle. *Development of Cost Analysis Reporting Forms and Procedures for a Medex Assisted Physician Practice.* Prepared by Stanford Research Institute, Menlo Park, Calif., for National Center for

Health Services Research and Development, Health Services and Mental Health Administration, U.S. Department of Health, Education and Welfare, Washington, D.C., January, 1971.

Haug, J. N., and B. C. Martin. *Foreign Medical Graduates in the United States, 1970.* Chicago: American Medical Association, 1971.

Haug, J. N., and G. A. Roback. *Distribution of Physicians, Hospitals, and Hospital Beds in the U.S., 1968: Regional, State, County, Metropolitan Area.* Chicago: American Medical Association, 1971.

———. *Distribution of Physicians, Hospitals, and Hospital Beds in the U.S., 1969,* vols. 1 and 2. Chicago: American Medical Association, 1970.

Haug, J. N., G. A. Roback, and B. C. Martin. *Distribution of Physicians in the United States, 1970: Regional State, County and Metropolitan Areas.* Chicago; American Medical Association, 1971.

Havighurst, Clark C., ed. *Health Care.* New York: Oceana Publications, 1972.

———. "Health Maintenance Organizations and the Market for Health Services." *Law and Contemporary Problems,* vol. 35 (Autumn 1970), pp. 716-95.

Health, Karen A., James K. Cooper, and Sinclair Coleman. *Choice of Location of Practice of Medical School Graduates: Analysis of Two Surveys,* R-1477-HEW. Santa Monica: The Rand Corporation, 1974.

Health Maintenance Organizations: A Reconfiguration of the Health Services System. Proceedings of the Thirteenth Annual Symposium on Hospital Affairs, University of Chicago, May 1971.

Heistand, Dale L. "Research into Manpower for Health Service." *Milbank Memorial Fund Quarterly,* vol. 44, no. 2 (October 1966), pp. 146-79.

Hendrickson, Robert M. "Physician Incomes. The Battle Against Inflation. Win, Lose or Draw?" *Prism* (May 1975), pp. 22-23, 59.

Hoffer, George E. "Physician Ownership in Pharmacies and Drug Repackers." *Inquiry,* vo. 12, no. 1 (March 1975), pp. 26-36.

Holtmann, Albert G. "Another Look at the Shortage of Physicians." *Industrial and Labor Relations Review,* vol. 18 (April 1965), pp. 423-24.

———. "Prices, Time, and Technology in the Medical Care Market." *Journal of Human Resources,* vol. 7, no. 2 (Spring 1972), pp. 179-90.

Human Resources Research Center, University of Southern California. *An Original Comparative Economic Analysis of Group Practice and Solo Fee-for-Service Practice: Final Report.* Prepared for National Center for Health Services Research, Springfield, Va., (PB 241 546), January 31, 1974.

Hyde, D. R., P. Wolff, Anne Gross, and E. L. Hoffmann. "The American Medical Association: Power, Purpose and Politics in Organized Medicine." *Yale Law Journal,* vol. 63 (May 1954), pp. 938-1022.

Hyman, Joseph, and Sherman Folland. "Uncertainty and Hospital Costs." *Southern Economic Journal,* vol. 39, no. 2 (October 1972), pp. 267-73.

Illich, Ivan. *Medical Nemesis.* London: Calder and Boyars, 1974.

Institute of Medicine. *Controls on Health Care.* Papers of the Conference on Regulation in the Health Industry, January 7-9, 1974. Washington, D.C.: National Academy of Sciences, 1975.

Intriligator, Michael D. "A Note on the Perceived Substitutability of Allied

Health Personnel for Selected Tasks in Physicians' Practice." In University of Southern California, Human Resources Research Center, *An Original Comparative Economic Analysis of Group Practice and Solo Fee-for-Service Practice: Final Report.* Prepared for National Center for Health Services Research, Springfield, Va., January 31, 1974.

Intriligator, Michael D., and Barbara H. Kehrer. "An Econometric Analysis of Employment and Utilization of Allied Health Personnel in Solo and Group Practices." In University of Southern California, Human Resources Research Center, *An Original Comparative Economic Analysis of Group Practice and Solo Fee-for-Service Practice: Final Report.* Prepared for National Center for Health Services Research, Springfield, Va., January 31, 1974.

Intriligator, Michael D., Richard Odem, Marianne Miller, and Herbert Schwartz, "Allied Health Personnel Hiring Sequence." In University of Southern California, Human Resource Research Center, *An Original Comparative Economic Analysis of Group Practice and Solo Fee-for-Service Practice: Final Report.* Prepared for National Center for Health Services Research, Springfield, Va., January 31, 1974.

"Is This Appendectomy Really Necessary?" *Medical World News* (March 10, 1975), pp. 21-22.

Jaco, E. Gartly, ed., *Patients, Physicians and Illness.* Glencoe, Ill.: The Free Press, 1958.

Jeffers, James R., Mario F. Bognanno, and John C. Bartlett. "On the Demand versus Need for Medical Services and the Concept of 'Shortage'." *American Journal of Public Health,* vol. 61 (January 1971), pp. 46-63.

Jeffers, William N. "Self-Employed M.D.s' Earnings and Expenses: How High the Bind?" *Medical Economics* (November 20, 1972), pp. 131-47.

Johnson, Sheila K. "My Doctor, the Corporation," *The New York Times Magazine* (December 29, 1974), pp. 8-9 and 18-21.

Joint Legislative Audit Committee, Office of the Auditor General, California Legislature. *Doctors' Malpractice Insurance,* Report 265.2. Sacramento, December 19, 1975.

Jones, Ellen W., Paul M. Densen, Isidore Altman, Sam Shapiro, and Howard West. "HIP Incentive Reimbursement Experiment: Utilization and Costs of Medical Care, 1969 and 1970." *Social Security Bulletin,* vol. 37 (December 1974), pp. 3-34.

Jones, Norman H., Jr., Charles A. Struve, and Paula Stefani. "Health Manpower in 1975—Demand, Supply, and Price." In U.S. National Advisory Commission on Health Manpower, *Report of the Commission,* vol. 2 (1967), pp. 229-63.

Kass, Leon R. "Regarding the End of Medicine and the Pursuit of Health." *The Public Interest,* no. 40 (Summer 1975), pp. 11-42.

Katz, Elihu. "The Social Itinerary of Technical Change: Two Studies on the Diffusion of Innovation." In Harper W. Boyd, Jr., and Joseph Newman, eds., *Advertising Management: Selected Readings.* Homewood, Ill.: Richard D. Irwin, 1965, p. 139.

Kehrer, Barbara H. "The Physician as Purchasing Agent for His Patient." In American Medical Association, *Socioeconomic Issues of Health and Medical Care.* Chicago: American Medical Association, 1974, pp. 55-61.

Kehrer, Barbara H., and Michael D. Intriligator, "Malpractice and the Employment of Allied Health Personnel." In University of Southern California, Human Resources Research Center, *An Original Comparative Economic Analysis of Group Practice and Solo Fee-for-Service Practice: Final Report.* Prepared for National Center for Health Services Research, Springfield, Va., January 31, 1974.

———. "Task Delegation in Physician Office Practice." In University of Southern California, Human Resources Research Center, *An Original Comparative Economic Analysis of Group Practice and Solo Fee-for-Service Practice: Final Report.* Prepared for National Center for Health Services Research, Springfield, Va., January 31, 1974.

Kehrer, Barbara H., and James C. Knowles, "Economies of Scale and the Pricing of Physicians' Services." In University of Southern California, Human Resources Research Center, *An Original Comparative Economic Analysis of Group Practice and Solo Fee-for-Service Practice: Final Report.* Prepared for National Center for Health Services Research, Springfield, Va., January 31, 1974.

Kessel, Reuben A. "Price Discrimination in Medicine." *Journal of Law and Economics*, vol. 1 (October 1958), pp. 20–54.

Kimbell, Larry J. "Dual Production, Cost and Factor Demand Function Estimation in an Errors-in-Variables Model." In University of Southern California, Human Resources Research Center, *An Original Comparative Economic Analysis of Group Practice and Solo Fee-for-Service Practice: Final Report.* Prepared for National Center for Health Services Research, Springfield, Va., January 31, 1974.

———. "Physician Behavior in Scarcity Areas." In University of Southern California, Human Resources Research Center, *An Original Comparative Economic Analysis of Group Practice and Solo Fee-for-Service Practice: Final Report.* Prepared for National Center for Health Services Research, Springfield, Va., January 31, 1974.

Kimbell, Larry J., and Robert T. Deane, "Analysis of the Utilization of Ancillary Personnel Using Production Functions." In University of Southern California, Human Resources Research Center, *An Original Comparative Economic Analysis of Group Practice and Solo Fee-for-Service Practice: Final Report.* Prepared for National Center for Health Services Research, Springfield, Va., January 31, 1974.

Kimbell, Larry J., and John H. Lorant, "Age-Income Patterns for Group and Solo Physicians." In University of Southern California, Human Resources Research Center, *An Original Comparative Economic Analysis of Group Practice and Solo Fee-for-Service Practice: Final Report.* Prepared for National Center for Health Services Research, Springfield, Va., January 31, 1974.

———. "Physician Productivity and Returns to Scale." In University of Southern California, Human Resources Research Center, *An Original Comparative Economic Analysis of Group Practice and Solo Fee-for-Service Practice: Final Report.* Prepared for National Center for Health Services Research, Springfield, Va., January 31, 1974.

———. "The Translog Production Function and the Substitution of Physicians,

Aides, and Capital." In University of Southern California, Human Resources Research Center, *An Original Comparative Economic Analysis of Group Practice and Solo Fee-for-Service Practice: Final Report*. Prepared for National Center for Health Services Research, Springfield, Va., January 31, 1974.

Kisch, Arnold I. "The Health Care System and Health: Some Thoughts on a Famous Misalliance." *Inquiry*, vol. 11, no. 4 (December 1974), pp. 269–75.

Kissick, William L., and Samuel P. Martin. "Issues of the Future in Health." *Annals of the American Academy of Political and Social Science*, vol. 399 (January 1972), pp. 151–59.

Klarman, Herbert E. "Analysis of the HMO Proposal—Its Assumptions, Implications, and Prospects." In *Health Maintenance Organizations: A Reconfiguration of the Health Services System*. Proceedings of the Thirteenth Annual Symposium on Hospital Affairs, Center for Health Administration Studies, University of Chicago, May 1971, pp. 24–38.

——. "Approaches to Moderating the Increases in Medical Care Costs," *Medical Care*, vol. 8 (May-June 1969), pp. 175–90.

——. "Economic Aspects of Projecting Requirements for Health Manpower." *Journal of Human Resources*, vol. 4 (1969), pp. 360–76.

——. "Major Public Initiatives in Health Care." *Public Interest*, no. 34 (Winter 1974), pp. 106–23.

——. *The Economics of Health*. New York: Columbia University Press, 1965.

Klaw, Spencer. *The Great American Medicine Show*. New York: The Viking Press, 1975.

Knowles, James C. "A Procedure for Estimating the Cost of Self-Employed Physician Labor." In University of Southern California, Human Resources Research Center, *An Original Comparative Economic Analysis of Group Practice and Solo Fee-for-Service Practice: Final Report*. Prepared for National Center for Health Services Research, Springfield, Va., January 31, 1974.

Knowles, John. "Where Doctors Fail." *Saturday Review* (August 22, 1970), pp. 21–23 and 63.

Kolodrubetz, Walter W. "Group Health Insurance Coverage of Full-Time Employees, 1972." *Social Security Bulletin*, vol. 37, no. 4 (April 1974), pp. 17–35.

Kovner, J.W. "A Production Function for Outpatient Medical Facilities." Unpublished Ph.D. dissertation, University of California, Los Angeles, 1968.

Lairson, Paul D., Jane C. Record, and Julia C. James. "Physician Assistants at Kaiser: Distinctive Patterns of Practice." *Inquiry*, vol. 11, no. 3 (September 1974), pp. 207–19.

Langendonck, Jozef Van. "The European Experience in Social Health Insurance." *Social Security Bulletin*, vol. 36, no. 7 (July 1973), pp. 27–30.

Lee, A. James, and Burton A. Weisbrod. "Collective Goods and the Voluntary Sector: The Case of the Hospital Industry." Center for Medical Sociology and Health Services Research, Health Economics Research Center, Research and Analytic Report Series. Madison: University of Wisconsin, July 1974.

Lee, Maw Lin. "A Conspicuous Production Theory of Hospital Behavior." *Southern Economic Journal*, vol. 38, no. 1 (July 1971), pp. 48–58.

Lee, Sidney S., and Lawrence M. Butler. "The Three-layered Cake—A Plan for Physician Compensation." *New England Journal of Medicine*, vol. 291, no. 5 (August 1, 1974), pp. 253-56.

Leibenstein, Harvey. "Allocative Efficiency vs. 'X-Efficiency'." *American Economic Review*, vol. 56 (June 1966), pp. 392-415.

——. "Competition and X-Efficiency," *Journal of Political Economy*, vol. 81 (May-June 1973), pp. 765-77.

Lembke, Paul A. "Medical Auditing by Scientific Methods. *Journal of the American Medical Association*, vol. 162, no. 7 (October 13, 1956), pp. 646-55.

Levitt, LeRoy P. "The Personality of the Medical Student." *Chicago Medical School Quarterly*, vol. 25, no. 4 (Winter 1966), pp. 201-14.

Lindsay, Cotton M., ed. *New Directions in Public Health Care: An Evaluation of Proposals for National Health Insurance*. San Francisco: Institute for Contemporary Studies, 1976.

——. "Real Returns to Medical Education." *Journal of Human Resources*, vol. 8, no. 3 (Summer 1973), pp. 331-48.

Litman, Theodor J. "Public Perceptions of the Physicians' Assistant—A Survey of the Attitudes and Opinions of Rural Iowa and Minnesota Residents." *American Journal of Public Health*, vol. 62 (March 1972), pp. 343-46.

Long, Hugh W., and J. B. Silvers. "Health Care Reimbursement is Federal Taxation of Tax-exempt Providers." *Health Care Management Review*, vol. 1, no. 1 (Winter 1975), pp. 9-23.

Lorant, John H., and Larry J. Kimbell. "Qualitative Determinants of Output in Group and Solo Medical Practice." In University of Southern California, Human Resources Research Center, *An Original Comparative Economic Analysis of Group Practice and Solo Fee-for-Service Practice: Final Report*. Prepared for National Center for Health Services Research, Springfield, Va., January 31, 1974.

MacColl, W. A. *Group Practice and Prepayment of Medical Care*. Washington, D. C.: Public Affairs Press, 1966.

MacLeod, Gordon K., and Jeffrey A. Prussing. "The Continuing Evolution of Health Maintenance Organizations." *New England Journal of Medicine*, vol. 288 (March 1, 1973).

Maddison, David. "Stress on the Doctor and His Family." *Medical Journal of Australia*, vol. 2 (August 31, 1974), pp. 315-23.

Mahoney, Anne R. "Factors Affecting Physicians' Choice of Group or Independent Practice." *Inquiry*, vol. 10, no. 2 (June 1973), pp. 9-18.

Massell, Adele P., and James R. Hosek. *Estimating the Effects of Teaching on the Costs of Inpatient Care: The Case of Radiology Treatments*, R-1751-HEW. Santa Monica, Calif.: The Rand Corporation, 1975.

McCarthy, Eugene G., and Geraldine W. Widmer. "Effects of Screening by Consultants on Recommended Elective Surgical Procedures," *New England Journal of Medicine*, vol. 291 (December 19, 1974), pp. 1331-35.

McKittrick. Leland S. "Rational Responses to Graduate Education of Physicians." *Journal of the American Medical Association*, vol. 201, no. 2 (July 10, 1967), pp. 112-14.

McNamara, Mary E., and Clifford Todd. "A Survey of Group Practice in the United States, 1969." *American Journal of Public Health*, vol. 60 (July 1970), pp. 1303-13.

McNeel, Richard, Jr., and Robert E. Schlenker. "HMOs, Competition, and Government." *Milbank Memorial Fund Quarterly, Health and Society*, vol. 53, no. 2 (Spring 1975), pp. 195-224.

McTaggart, Aubrey C. *The Health Care Dilemma.* Boston: Holbrook Press, 1971.

Mechanic, David. "Human Problems and the Organization of Health Care." *Annals of the American Academy of Political and Social Science*, vol. 399 (January 1972), pp. 1-11.

——. "Problems in the Future Organization of Medical Practice." *Law and Contemporary Problems*, vol. 35, no. 2 (Spring 1970), pp. 54-58.

Medical Economics. *First Steps Toward Private Medical Practice.* Oradell, N.J.: Medical Economics Book Division, Inc., 1965.

——. *Tax-Savings Guide for Physicians.* Oradell, N.J.: Medical Economics Book Division, Inc., 1967.

"Medical Inflation Goes Under the Knife." *Business Week* (April 4, 1970), pp. 26-27.

Meeker, Edward. "Allocation of Resources to Health Revisited." *Journal of Human Resources*, vol. 8, no. 2 (Spring 1973), pp. 257-59.

Mitchell, Bridger M., and Charles E. Phelps. *Employer-paid Group Health Insurance and the Costs of Mandated National Coverage*, R-1509-HEW. Santa Monica, Calif.: The Rand Corporation, 1975.

Mitchell, Bridger M., and William B. Schwartz. *The Financing of National Health Insurance*, R-1711-HEW. Santa Monica, Calif.: The Rand Corporation, 1976.

Modlin, Herbert C., and Alberto Montes. "Narcotics Addiction in Physicians." *American Journal of Psychiatry* (October 1964), pp. 358-65.

Monsma, George N., Jr. "Marginal Revenue and the Demand for Physicians' Services." In Herbert E. Klarman, ed., *Empiricial Studies in Health Economics.* Proceedings of the Second Conference on the Economics of Health. Baltimore, Md.: The Johns Hopkins Press, 1970.

——. "The Supply of and Demand for Physicians' Services." Unpublished Ph.D. Dissertation, Princeton University, Princeton, N.J., 1969.

Morreale, Joseph C., ed. *The U.S. Medical Care Industry: The Economist's Point of View*, Michigan Business Papers Number 60. Ann Arbor: Division of Research, Graduate School of Business Administration, University of Michigan, 1974.

Mueller, Marjorie S. "Private Health Insurance in 1972: Health Care Services, Enrollment, and Finances." *Social Security Bulletin*, vol. 37, no. 2 (February 1974), pp. 20-40.

——. "Private Health Insurance in 1973: A Review of Coverage, Enrollment, and Financial Experience." *Social Security Bulletin*, vol. 38, no. 2 (February 1975), pp. 21-40.

Mueller, Marjorie S., and Robert M. Gibson. "Age Differences in Health Care Spending, Fiscal Year 1974." *Social Security Bulletin*, vol. 38, no. 6 (June 1975), pp. 3-16.

——. "National Health Expenditures, Fiscal Year 1975." *Social Security Bulletin*, vol. 39, no. 2 (February 1976).

Mueller, Marjorie S., and Paula A. Piro. "Private Health Insurance in 1974: A Review of Coverage, Enrollment, and Financial Experience." *Social Security Bulletin*, vol. 39, no. 3 (March 1976), pp. 3–20.

Mumford, Emily. *Interns: From Students to Physicians.* Cambridge, Mass.: Harvard University Press, 1970.

National Advisory Commission on Health Manpower. *The Kaiser Foundation Medical Care Program.* Special reprint of Vol. II, Appendix IV, pp. 197–228, National Advisory Commission on Health Manpower, *Report of the Commission*, 2 vols. Washington, D.C.: U.S. Government Printing Office, 1967.

National Opinion Research Center. *Career Preferences of Medical Students in the United States.* Study in Conjunction with Office of the Surgeon General, Department of the Army, Publication No. DA 4900719. Chicago, 1956.

Nelson, Eugene C., Arthur R. Jacobs, and Kenneth G. Johnson. "Patients' Acceptance of Physician Assistants." *Journal of the American Medical Association*, vol. 228, no. 1 (April 1, 1974), pp. 63–67.

Neuhauser, Duncan, and William Halperin. *Cost-Effective Clinical Decision Making.* Cases in Health Service Series No. 3B. Boston: Harvard School of Public Health and Center for Community Health and Medical Care, 1973.

Neuhauser, Duncan, and A. M. Lewicki. "National Health Insurance and the Sixth Stool Guaiac." *Policy Analysis*, vol. 2, no. 2 (Spring 1976), pp. 175–96.

Newhouse, Joseph P. "A Model of Physician Pricing." *Southern Economic Journal*, vol. 37, no. 2 (October 1970), pp. 174–83.

——. "The Economics of Group Practice." *Journal of Human Resources*, vol. 8, no. 1 (Winter 1973), pp. 37–56.

Newhouse, Joseph P., Charles E. Phelps, and William B. Schwartz. "Policy Options and the Impact of National Health Insurance." *New England Journal of Medicine*, vol. 290 (June 13, 1974), pp. 1345–59.

Newhouse, Joseph P., and Frank A. Sloan. "Physician Pricing: Monopolistic or Competitive: Comment." *Southern Economic Journal*, vol. 38, no. 4 (April 1972), pp. 573–80.

——. "Physician Pricing: Monopolistic or Competitive: Reply." *Southern Economic Journal*, vol. 38, no. 4 (April 1972), pp. 577–80.

Newhouse, Joseph P., and Vincent Taylor. "The Subsidy Problem in Hospital Insurance: A Proposal." *Journal of Business*, vol. 48 (October 1970), pp. 452–56.

Noll, Roger G. "The Consequences of Public Regulation of Hospitals." Paper delivered to the Institute of Medicine Conference on Regulation in the Health Industry, Washington, D.C., January 1974.

Notes and Brief Reports. "Prescription Drugs, 1967–71." *Social Security Bulletin*, vol. 37, no. 2 (February 1974), pp. 41–45.

——. "Rhode Island Catastrophic Health Insurance Plan." *Social Security Bulletin*, vol. 38, no. 2 (February 1975), pp. 41–43.

Ostergard, Donald R., Elmer M. Broen, and John R. Marshall. "The Family Planning Specialist as a Provider of Health Care Services." *Fertility and Sterility*, vol. 23, no. 7 (July 1972), pp. 505–07.

Ostergard, Donald R., John E. Gunning, and John R. Marshall. "Training and Function of a Women's Health-Care Specialist, or Nurse Practitioner in Obstetrics and Gynecology." *American Journal of Obstetrics and Gynecology*, vol. 121, no. 8 (April 15, 1975), pp. 1029-37.

Otis, Gerald D., and Joann R. Weiss. "Patterns of Medical Career Preference." *Journal of Medical Education*, vol. 48 (December 1973), pp. 1116-23.

"Overmanagement of Medicine." *Science*, vol. 183, no. 4121 (January 18, 1974).

Owens, Arthur. "After the Freeze. . . Can Self-Employed M.D.s Break Out?" *Medical Economics* (November 11, 1974), pp. 232-40.

――. "General Surgeons: Too Many in the Wrong Places." *Medical Economics* (July 20, 1973), pp. 128-33.

――. "How Do Your Practice Goals Compare?" *Medical Economics* (February 20, 1967), pp. 65-73.

――. "How Many Doctors Are Really Working at Full Capacity?" *Medical Economics* (January 18, 1971), pp. 85-93.

――. "Inflation Closes in on Physicians' Earnings." *Medical Economics* (December 21, 1970), pp. 63-71.

――. "Physicians' Earnings: Leveling Off." *Medical Economics* (October 11, 1971), pp. 203-11.

――. "Practice Costs: How High Will They Go?" *Medical Economics* (November 23, 1970), pp. 81-91.

――. "Raise Fees After the Freeze? Think Twice!" *Medical Economics* (November 8, 1971), pp. 189-97.

――. "The Economics of Partnership Practice." *Medical Economics* (June 12, 1967), pp. 86-95.

――. "The New Surge in Physicians' Earnings and Expenses." *Medical Economics* (December 8, 1969, pp. 83-89.

――. "Time Well Spent? New Norms Will Help You See." *Medical Economics* (December 6, 1971), pp. 79-87.

――. "Your Lifetime Earnings: How Much Will You Keep?" *Medical Economics* (November 22, 1971), pp. 81-84.

Page, Robert G., and Mary H. Littlemeyer. *Preparation for the Study of Medicine*. Chicago: The University of Chicago Press, 1969.

Parker, Harry J., and John C. Delahunt. "Delegating Tasks to Physicians' Assistants: Physicians' Reactions." *Texas Medicine*, vol. 68 (October 1972), pp. 69-79.

Pauly, Mark V. "Efficiency, Incentives and Reimbursement for Health Care." *Inquiry*, vol. 7 (March 1970), pp. 114-31.

Pauly, Mark V., and M. Redisch. "The Not-For-Profit Hospital as a Physicians Cooperative." *American Economic Review*, vol. 63, no. 1 (March 1973), pp. 87-99.

Paxton, Harry T., and David Whieldon. "A Doctor's Guide to Practice Management Consultants." *Medical Economics* (December 4, 1972), pp. 111-61.

Pearson, Manuel M., and Edward A. Strecher. "Physicians as Psychiatric Patients: Private Practice Experience." *American Journal of Psychiatry* (April 1960), pp. 915-19.

Peel, Evelyn, and Jack Scharff. "Impact of Cost-Sharing on Use of Ambulatory Services Under Medicare, 1969." *Social Security Bulletin,* vol. 36 (October 1973), pp. 3–24.

Perlman, Mark, ed. *The Economics of Health and Medical Care: Proceedings of a Conference Held by the International Economic Association at Tokyo.* New York: John Wiley and Sons, 1974.

Perrott, George S. "The Federal Employees Health Benefits Program." *Group Health and Welfare News* (Special Supplement, March 21, 1971).

——. "Utilization of Hospital Services." *American Journal of Public Health,* vol. 56 (January 1966), pp. 57–64.

Perrott, George S., and Maryland Y. Pennell. "Physician Shortage Reconsidered." *New England Journal of Medicine,* vol. 275 (July 14, 1966), pp. 85–87.

——. "Physicians in the United States: Projections 1955–1975." *Journal of Medical Education,* vol. 33 (September 1958), pp. 638–44.

Peterson, Paul Q., and Maryland Y. Pennell. "Physician Population Projections, 1961–75: Their Causes and Implications." *American Journal of Public Health,* vol. 53 (February 1963), pp. 163–72.

Pettengill, Julian. "The Financial Position of Private Community Hospitals, 1961–71." *Social Security Bulletin,* vol. 36, no. 11 (November 1973), pp. 3–19.

Phelps, Charles E., and Joseph P. Newhouse. "Coinsurance, the Price of Time, and the Demand for Medical Services." *Review of Economics and Statistics,* vol. 56, no. 3 (August 1974), pp. 334–42.

Powell, J. Enoch. *Medicine and Politics.* London: Pitman Medical Publishing Co., 1966.

Promoting the Group Practice of Medicine. Report of the National Conference on Group Practice, October, 1967. Washington, D.C.: U.S. Government Printing Office, 1967.

Rayack, Elton. *Professional Power and American Medicine: The Economics of the American Medical Association.* Cleveland: World Publishing Co., 1967.

——. "The Physician's Service Industry." In Walter Adams, *The Structure of American Industry,* 4th ed. New York: Macmillan, 1971, pp. 419–56.

——. "The Shortage of Physician Services." *Industrial and Labor Relations Review,* vol. 18 (July 1965), pp. 584–87.

——. "The Supply of Physician Services." *Industrial and Labor Relations Review,* vol. 17 (January 1964), pp. 221–37.

Record, Jane C., Joan E. O'Bannon, Paul D. Lairson, and John P. Mullooly. "Cost Effectiveness of Physician's Associates: Kaiser-Permanente Experience." Presented at Meetings of the Health Economics Research Organization Dallas, December 1975.

Reder, Melvin W. "Some Problems in the Measurement of Productivity in Medical Care Industry." In Victor R. Fuchs, ed., *Production and Productivity in the Service Industries.* Prepared for National Bureau of Economic Research, Studies in Income and Wealth. New York: Columbia University Press, 1969.

Reinhardt, Uwe E. "Alternative Methods of Reimbursing Non-Institutional

Providers of Health Services." Paper presented to the Institute of Medicine Conference on Regulation in the Health Industry, National Academy of Sciences, Washington, D.C., January 1974.

————. "An Economic Analysis of Physicians' Practices." Unpublished Ph.D. Dissertation, Yale University, New Haven, Conn., 1970.

————. "A Production Function for Physician Services," *Review of Economics and Statistics*, vol. 54, no. 1 (February 1972), pp. 55–66.

————. "Manpower Substitution and Productivity in Medical Practice: Review of Research." *Health Services Research* (Fall 1973).

————. *Physician Productivity and the Demand for Health Manpower, An Economic Analysis*. Cambridge, Mass.: Ballinger Publishing Company, 1975.

————. "Proposed Changes in the Organization of Health-Care Delivery: An Overview and Critique." *Milbank Memorial Fund Quarterly, Health and Society*, vol. 51, no. 2 (Spring 1973), pp. 169–222.

Reinhardt, Uwe E., and Donald E. Yett. "Physician Production Functions Under Varying Practice Arrangements," Technical Paper No. 11. Community Profile Data Center, August 1972.

Riddick. Frank A., John B. Bryan, Maurice I. Gershenson, and Addis C. Costello. "Use of Allied Health Professionals in Internists' Offices." *Archives of Internal Medicine*, vol. 127 (May 1971), pp. 924–31.

Rimlinger, Gaston V., and Henry B. Steele. "An Economic Interpretation of the Spatial Distribution of Physicians in the U.S." *Southern Economic Journal*, vol. 30 (July 1963), pp. 1–12.

Roback, G. A., ed. *Distribution of Physicians in the United States, 1971*. Chicago: American Medical Association, 1972.

Robbins, Anthony. "The Physician's Voice in Hospital Management." *Monthly Labor Review*, vol. 94, no. 4 (April 1971), pp. 60–62.

Roemer, Milton I. "On Paying the Doctor and the Implications of Different Methods." *Journal of Health and Human Behavior*, vol. 3 (Spring 1962), pp. 10–19.

Roemer, Milton I., and Donald M. DuBois. "Medical Costs in Relation to the Organization of Ambulatory Care." *New England Journal of Medicine*, vol. 280, no. 18 (May 1, 1969), pp. 988–93.

Roemer, Milton I., Robert W. Hetherington, Carl E. Hopkins, Arthur E. Gerst, Eleanor Parsons, and Donald M. Long. *Health Insurance Effects: Services, Expenditures, and Attitudes Under Three Types of Plans*, Bureau of Public Health Economics Research Series No. 16. Ann Arbor: School of Public Health, University of Michigan, 1972.

Roemer, Milton I., and William Shonick. "HMO Performance: The Recent Evidence." *Milbank Memorial Fund Quarterly, Health and Society*, vol. 51, no. 3 (Summer 1973), pp. 271–317.

Roos, N. P. "Influencing the Health Care System: Policy Alternatives." *Public Policy*, vol. 22, no. 2 (Spring 1974), pp. 139–67.

Rose, K. Daniel. "Physicians Who Kill Themselves." *Archives of General Psychiatry*, vol. 29 (December 1973), pp. 800–05.

Rosenberg, M. *Occupations and Values*. New York: The Free Press of Glencoe, 1957.

Rosenthal, Neal H. "The Health Manpower Gap: A High Hurdle." *Occupational Outlook Quarterly*, vol. 2 (February 1967).

Rosett, Richard N., ed. *The Role of Health Insurance in the Health Services Sector*. Prepared for National Bureau of Economic Research. New York: Neale Watson Academic Publications, 1976.

Rosett, Richard N., and Lein-fu Huang. "The Effect of Health Insurance on the Demand for Medical Care." *Journal of Political Economy*, vol. 81, no. 2, Part 1 (March-April 1973), pp. 281-305.

Rucker, T. Donald. "Economic Problems in Drug Distribution." *Inquiry*, vol. 9, no. 3 (September 1972), pp. 43-50.

Ruffin, Roy J., and Duane E. Leigh. "Charity, Competition, and the Pricing of Doctors' Services." *Journal of Human Resources*, vol. 8, no. 2 (Fall 1972), pp. 212-22.

Ruhe, C. H. William. "Present Projections of Physician Production." *Journal of the American Medical Association*, vol. 193 (December 5, 1966), pp. 1094-1100.

Russe, J. "The Use and Abuse of Laboratory Tests." *Medical Clinics of North America*, vol. 53 (1969), pp. 223-31.

Sadler, Alfred M., Jr., Blair L. Sadler, and Ann A. Bliss. *The Physician's Assistant Today and Tomorrow*. New Haven, Conn.: Yale University School of Medicine, 1972.

Scaer, Robert C. "There's a Doctor Surplus in our Town. Will Yours be Next?" *Medical Economics* (September 3, 1973), pp. 81-84.

Scheffler, Richard M. "The Pricing Behavior of Medical Groups." *Milbank Memorial Fund Quarterly, Health and Society*, vol. 53, no. 2 (Spring 1975), pp. 225-40.

Schulz, Rockwell I., and Jerry Rose. "Can Hospitals Be Expected to Control Costs?" *Inquiry*, vol. 10, no. 2 (June 1973), pp. 3-8.

Schumer, Rona B. "Hospital Utilization Review and Medicare: A Survey," U.S. Department of Health, Education, and Welfare, Social Security Administration, Office of Research and Statistics, Staff Paper No. 8. Washington, D.C., 1971.

Schwartz, Harry. *The Case for American Medicine: A Realistic Look at our Health Care System*. New York: David McKay Company, 1972.

Schwartz, Herbert J. "Application of Cluster Analysis to Estimation of Cost Functions for Group Medical Practice." In University of Southern California, Human Resources Research Center, *An Original Comparative Economic Analysis of Group Practice and Solo Fee-for-Service Practice: Final Report*. Prepared for National Center for Health Services Research, Springfield, Va., January 31, 1974.

Schwartz, Herbert J., and Richard L. Ernst. "Cobb-Douglas and Constant-Elasticity-of-Substitution Cost Functions for Physicians' Practices." In University of Southern California, Human Resources Research Center, *An Original Comparative Economic Analysis of Group Practice and Solo Fee-for-Service Practice: Final Report*. Prepared for National Center for Health Services Research, Springfield, Va., January 31, 1974.

Schwartz, William B. "Medicine and the Computer: The Promise and Problems of Change." *New England Journal of Medicine*, vol. 283 (December 1970), pp. 1257–64.

———. Testimony in *Hearings* before the Subcommittee on Health of the Committee on Labor and Public Welfare, U.S. Senate, 92nd Congress, First Session, on Examination of the Health Care Crisis in America, Part 3, pp. 442–62. Washington, D.C.: U.S. Government Printing Office, May 10, 1971.

Scitovsky, Anne A. "Changes in the Costs of Treatment of Selected Illnesses, 1951–1965." *American Economic Review*, vol. 57 (December 1967).

Scitovsky, Anne A., and Nelda McCall. "Changes in the Costs of Treatment of Selected Illnesses, 1951–1964–1971," Discussion Paper. San Francisco: Health Policy Program, University of California, September 1975.

Scott, Charles D. "Health Care Delivery and Advanced Technology." *Science*, vol. 180 (June 29, 1973), pp. 1339–42.

Sgontz, Larry G. "The Economics of Financing Medical Care: A Review of the Literature." *Inquiry*, vol. 9, no. 4 (December 1972), pp. 3–19.

Shapiro, Edith T., Henry Pinsker, and John H. Shale. "The Mentally Ill Physician as Practitioner." *Journal of the American Medical Association*, vol. 232 (May 19, 1975), pp. 725–27.

Silverman, Milton, and Philip R. Lee. *Pills, Profits, and Politics.* Berkeley: University of California Press, 1974.

Skipper, James D., Jr., Gary Smith, Jack L. Mulligan, and Mohan L. Garg. "Physicians' Knowledge of Cost: The Case of Diagnostic Tests." *Inquiry*, vol. 13, no. 2 (June 1976), pp. 194–98.

Sloan, Frank A. "A Microanalysis of Physicians' Hours of Work Decisions." Paper presented at the International Economic Association Conference of Health and Medical Care, Tokyo, 1973.

———. "Effect of Incentives on Physician Practice Performance." In John Rafferty, ed., *Health Manpower and Productivity.* Lexington, Mass.: D. C. Heath, 1974.

———. "Lifetime Earnings and the Physicians' Choice of Specialty." *Industrial and Labor Relations Review*, vol. 24 (1970), pp. 47–56.

———. "Physician Fee Inflation: Evidence from the late 1960's." Paper presented at the National Bureau of Economic Research Conference on the Role of Health Insurance in the Health Services Sector, Rochester, N.Y., May 1974.

———. *Supply Responses of Young Physicians: An Analysis of Physicians in Residency Programs.* Santa Monica, Calif: The Rand Corporation, 1973.

Sloan, Frank A., and Bruce Steinwald. "The Role of Health Insurance in the Physicians' Services Market." *Inquiry*, vol. 12, no. 4 (December 1975), pp. 275–99.

Small, Iver F., Joyce G. Small, Calre M. Assue, and Donald F. Moore. "The Fate of the Mentally Ill Physician." *American Journal of Psychiatry*, vol. 125 (April 10, 1969), pp. 1333–42.

Smith, Beverly. "Diagnosing the Doctors." *The Reader's Digest*, vol. 33, no. 196 (August 1938), pp. 1–5.

Smith, Kenneth R., Marianne Miller, and Frederick L. Golladay. "An Analysis of the Optimal Use of Inputs in the Production of Medical Services." *Journal of Human Resources*, vol. 7, no. 2 (Spring 1972), pp. 208–25.

Smith, Waverly G. "The Malpractice Crisis and the Insurance Carrier." *Transactions of the American Academy of Ophthalmology and Otolaryngology*, vol. 80, No. 3 (May-June 1975), pp. 286-90.

Smothers, David. "AMA Seeks Cure for Its Own Ailments—Indifference, Defections, Lack of Funds." *Los Angeles Times* (Sunday, April 27, 1975), Part 1.

Somers, Anne R. *Health Care in Transition: Directions for the Future.* Chicago: Hospital Research and Educational Trust, 1971.

——, ed. *The Kaiser-Permanente Medical Care Program: A Symposium.* New York: The Commonwealth Fund, 1971.

Somers, Harold M., and Anne R. Somers. *Doctors, Patients and Health Insurance.* Washington, D.C.: The Brookings Institution, 1961.

Somers, Herman M. "Health and Public Policy." *Inquiry*, vol. 12, no. 2 (June 1975), pp. 87-96.

Sorkin, Alan L. *Health Economics.* Lexington, Mass.: Lexington Books, 1975.

Spiegel, Allen D., and Simon Podair, eds. *Medicaid: Lessons for National Health Insurance.* Rockville, Md.: Aspen Systems Corporation, 1975.

Starr, Paul. "The Undelivered Health System." *The Public Interest* (Winter 1976), pp. 66-85.

Steinwald, Bruce, and Frank A. Sloan. "Determinants of Physicians' Fees." *Journal of Business*, vol. 47, no. 4 (October 1974), pp. 493-511.

Steinwald, C. "Factors Influencing the Distribution and Location of Physicians: Literature Review." In Roback, G. A., ed., *Distribution of Physicians in the United States.* Chicago: American Medical Association, 1972.

Stevens, Carl M. "Physician Supply and National Health Goals." *Journal of Industrial Relations*, vol. 10 (May 1971), pp. 119-44.

Stevens, Rosemary. *American Medicine and the Public Interest.* New Haven, Conn.: Yale University Press, 1971.

Stewart, Charles T., Jr., and Corazon M. Siddayao. *Increasing the Supply of Medical Personnel: Needs and Alternatives.* Washington, D.C.: American Enterprise Institute for Public Policy Research, 1973.

Stigler, George J. "The Xistence of X-Efficiency." *American Economic Review*, vol. 66, no. 1 (March 1976), pp. 213-16.

"Still Waiting for that Revolutionary Health Plan." *Business Week* (January 13, 1975), pp. 53-54.

"Symposium: Physician Productivity and the Hospital." *Inquiry*, vol. 6, no. 3 (September 1969), pp. 57-78.

Terasawa, Katsuaki, and David Whipple. *On the Comparative Costing of Military vs. Civilian Modes of Health Care Delivery.* Prepared for Bureau of Medicine and Surgery, Washington, D.C. Monterey, Calif.: Naval Postgraduate School, November 1975.

Terman, Lewis M. "Scientists and Nonscientists in a Group of 800 Gifted Men." *Psychological Monographs: General and Applied*, vol. 68, no. 7, whole no. 378, 1954.

The Conference Board. *Industry Roles in Health Care.* New York: The Conference Board, 1974.

The Economics of Health and Medical Care. Proceedings of the Conference on the Economics of Health and Medical Care, May 10-12, 1962. Sponsored by

Bureau of Public Health Economics and Department of Economics, University of Michigan, Ann Arbor, 1964.

"The HMO Movement Stalls Once More." *Business Week* (April 21, 1975), p. 31.

"Their First Year of Practice." *Medical Economics* (February 5, 1973), pp. 150–58.

Theodore, Christ N., and James N. Haug. *Selected Characteristics of the Physician Population, 1963 and 1967.* Chicago: American Medical Association, 1968.

Theodore, Christ N., and Gerald E. Sutter. "A Report on the First Periodic Survey of Physicians." *Journal of the American Medical Association*, vol. 202, no. 6 (November 6, 1967), pp. 516–24.

"The Sky's the Limit on Health Care Costs." *Business Week* (May 26, 1975), pp. 72–74.

Thompson, Theodis. "Selected Characteristics of Black Physicians in the United States, 1972." *Journal of the American Medical Association*, vol. 299, no. 13 (September 23, 1974), pp. 1758–61.

Todd, C., and M. E. McNamara. *Medical Groups in the U.S., 1969.* Chicago: American Medical Association, 1971.

Todd, Malcolm C. "Medical Manpower and the Emergence of New Professions." *Texas Medicine*, vol. 68 (October 1972), pp. 60–64.

Todd, Malcolm C., and Donald F. Foy. "Current Status of the Physician's Assistant and Related Issues." *Journal of the American Medical Association*, vol. 220 (June 26, 1972), pp. 1714–20.

Townes, C. Dwight. "the Doctor's Image of Himself." *Minnesota Medicine* (April 1974), pp. 315–18.

Tucker, Murray. "Utilization and Price Analysis: Prospects for Avoiding Higher Program Costs in Health Care." *American Journal of Public Health*, vol. 59, no. 7 (July 1969).

U.S. Congress, House Subcommittee on Public Health and Environment, Committee on Interstate and Foreign Commerce. *Hearings on the Health Professions Educational Assistance Amendments of 1971*, Parts 1 and 2, 92nd Congress, 1st Session, Washington, D.C., April 2–29, 1971.

U.S. Department of Health, Education and Welfare, Office of the Secretary, *Medical Care Prices, A Report to the President* (also referred to as the "Gorham Report"). Washington, D.C.: U.S. Government Printing Office, 1967.

U.S. Department of Health, Education and Welfare. *Report of the Secretary's Commission on Medical Malpractice*, DHEW Publication No. (OS) 73-88. Washington, D.C., January 16, 1973.

Vaillant, George E., Nancy C. Sobowale, and Charles McArthur. "Some Psychologic Vulnerabilities of Physicians." *New England Journal of Medicine*, vol. 287, no. 8 (August 24, 1972), pp. 372–75.

Vogel, Ronald J., and Roger D. Blair. *Health Insurance Administrative Costs*, U.S. Department of Health, Education and Welfare, Social Security Administration, Office of Research and Statistics, DHEW Publication No. (SSA) 76-11856, Staff Paper No. 21. Washington, D.C.: U.S. Government Printing Office, 1975.

Ward, Richard A. *The Economics of Health Resources*. Reading, Mass.: Addison-Wesley Publishing Company, 1975.

Warren, David G., and Richard Merritt, eds. *A Legislator's Guide to the Medical Malpractice Issue*. Washington, D.C.: Georgetown University, 1976.

Warshaw, Leon J. "The HMO Concept and Its Current Status." *Journal of Occupational Medicine*, vol. 17, no. 10 (October 1975), pp. 630–35.

Weinberger, Casper W. "Malpractice—A National View." *Arizona Medicine*, vol. 32, no. 2 (February 1975), pp. 117–18.

Weinerman, E. R. "Research into the Organization of Medical Practice." *Milbank Memorial Fund Quarterly*, vol. 63 (October 1966), pp. 117–18.

Weiss, Jeffrey H. "A Proposal for Financing the Purchase of Health Services: A Comment." *Journal of Human Resources*, vol. 6, no. 1 (Winter 1971), pp. 75–102.

———. "The Changing Job Structure of Health Manpower." Unpublished Ph.D. Dissertation, Harvard University, Cambridge, Mass., 1966.

Weiss, Jeffrey H., and Lynda Brodsky. "An Essay on the National Financing of Health Care." *Journal of Human Resources*, vol. 7, no. 2 (Spring 1972), pp. 139–51.

Wersinger, Richard, Klaus J. Roughmann, J. William Gavett, and Sandra M. Wells. "Inpatient Hospital Utilization in Three Prepaid Comprehensive Health Care Plans Compared with a Regular Blue Cross Plan." *Medical Care*, vol. 14, no. 9 (September 1976), pp. 721–32.

"What Controls Mean to Medical Care." *Business Week* (January 1, 1972), pp. 38–39.

Whieldon, David. "What Doctors Are Doing About Raising Aides' Pay." *Medical Economics* (December 7, 1970), pp. 99–129.

Willcox, Alanson W. "Hospitals and the Corporate Practice of Medicine." *Cornell Law Quarterly*, vol. 43 (1960), pp. 432–87.

Williams, Kathleen N., and Robert H. Brook. *Foreign Medical Graduates and Their Effects on the Quality of Medical Care in the United States*, R-1698-HEW. Santa Monica, Calif.: The Rand Corporation, 1976.

Wilson, Florence A., and Duncan Neuhauser. *Health Services in the United States*. Cambridge, Mass.: Ballinger Publishing Company, 1974.

Wilson, V. L., ed. *Medical School Admission Requirements, 1975–76, U.S.A. and Canada*. Washington, D.C.: Association of American Medical Colleges, 1974.

Wolfe, Sidney M. Testimony in *Hearings* before the Subcommittee on Oversight and Investigations on Unnecessary Surgery of the Interstate and Foreign Commerce Committee, House of Representatives, 94th Congress, 1st Session, Washington, D.C., July 15, 1975.

Worthington, Nancy L. "Expenditures for Hospital Care and Physicians' Services: Factors Affecting Annual Changes." *Social Security Bulletin*, vol. 38, no. 11 (November 1975), pp. 3–15.

———. "National Health Expenditures, 1929–74." *Social Security Bulletin*, vol. 38 (February 1975), pp. 3–20.

Yankauer, Alfred, John P. Connelly, and Jacob J. Feldman. "Physician Productivity in the Delivery of Ambulatory Care: Some Findings from a Survey of Pediatricians." *Medical Care*, vol. 8 (January-February 1970), pp. 35-46.

——. "Task Performance and Task Delegation in Pediatric Office Practice." *American Journal of Public Health*, vol. 59 (July 1969), pp. 1104-17.

Yankauer, Alfred, Sally H. Jones, Jan Schneider, and Louis M. Hellmann. "Performance and Delegation of Patient Services by Physicians in Obstetrics-Gynecology." *American Journal of Public Health*, vol. 61 (August 1971), pp. 1545-55.

Yankauer, Alfred, Jan Schneider, Sally H. Jones, Louis M. Hellmann, and Jacob J. Feldman. "Physician Output, Productivity and Task Delegation in Obstetrics-Gynecologic Practices in the United States." *Obstetrics and Gynecology*, vol. 39, no. 1 (January 1972), pp. 151-61.

Yett, Donald E. "An Evaluation of Alternative Methods of Estimating Physicians' Expenses Relative to Output." *Inquiry*, vol. 4, no. 1 (March 1967), pp. 3-27.

Yost, Edward. *The U.S. Health Industry: The Costs of Acceptable Medical Care by 1975.* New York: Praeger, 1969.

Zeckhauser, Richard, and Michael Eliastam. "The Productivity Potential of the Physician Assistant." *Journal of Human Resources*, vol. 9, no. 1 (Winter 1974), pp. 95-116.

Index

About the Authors

Joseph LaDou, M.D., trained at Harvard University and at the University of California. He is certified by the American Board of Preventive Medicine. For the past twelve years he has practiced medicine in the San Francisco Bay Area. As the senior partner in a medical group, he has witnessed firsthand many of the problems discussed in this book. Dr. LaDou's involvement as chairman of the San Mateo County Board of Health and Welfare provides further background. Since 1968 he has been a consultant to the Stanford Research Institute. Dr. LaDou has published numerous articles in scientific journals on preventive medicine and health care economics.

James D. Likens is Associate Professor of Economics at Pomona College. He obtained the B.A. and M.B.A. degrees from the University of California at Berkeley and the Ph.D. in economics from the University of Minnesota. His research interests involve topics in industrial organization and antitrust, transportation, and health economics. Professor Likens has had extensive experience as a consultant to private industry.

The authors met in 1969 at the request of a large manufacturing firm interested in finding ways to diversify into the medical products industry. Their continued interest in the economics of health care brings them together again in the publication of *Medicine and Money: Physicians as Businessmen.*

Date Due

NO2 5 '96		